# CONTINUITY IN PALLIATIVE CARE

# CONTINUITY IN PALLIATIVE CARE

## KEY ISSUES AND PERSPECTIVES

*Edited by Dan Munday and Cathy Shipman*

ROYAL COLLEGE OF GENERAL PRACTITIONERS

The Royal College of General Practitioners was founded
in 1952 with this object:

*'To encourage, foster and maintain the highest possible standards
in general practice and for that purpose to take or join with others
in taking steps consistent with the charitable nature of that object
which may assist towards the same.'*

Among its responsibilities under its Royal Charter the
College is entitled to:

*'Diffuse information on all matters affecting general practice and
issue such publications as may assist the object of the College.'*

**British Library Cataloguing-in-Publication Data**
**A catalogue record for this book is available from the British Library**

©Royal College of General Practitioners, 2007
Published by the Royal College of General Practitioners, 2007
14 Princes Gate, Hyde Park, London sw7 1pu

**Disclaimer**
This publication is intended for the use of medical practitioners in the UK
and not for patients. The authors, editors and publisher have taken care to
ensure that the information contained in this book is correct to the best of their
knowledge, at the time of publication. Whilst efforts have been made to ensure
the accuracy of the information presented, particularly that related to the
prescription of drugs, the authors, editors and publisher cannot accept liability
for information that is subsequently shown to be wrong. Readers are advised
to check that the information, especially that related to drug usage, complies
with information contained in the *British National Formulary*, or equivalent,
or manufacturers' datasheets, and that it complies with the latest legislation
and standards of practice.

Designed and typeset at the Typographic Design Unit

Printed by Latimer Trend

Indexed by Carol Ball

ISBN 978-0-85084-311-8

# Contents

# Foreword

I was honoured and delighted to receive an invitation from Dan
Munday and Cathy Shipman to write the Foreword to this book
published by the Royal College of General Practitioners. I am particularly pleased that they chose continuity of care as the title and underlying theme. As outlined in Chapter 1, it is perhaps no accident that
the topic of continuity of care was one of the earliest ones addressed
by the NHS Service Delivery and Organisation Research and Development (SDO) Programme. Work on the theme started with a scoping study to look at the meaning of the concept of 'continuity of care'
by examining the relevant literature. This scoping study by Professor
George Freeman *et al.* in 2000 concluded that continuity of care is a
multi-faceted concept used in a series of different ways including:
continuity across organisational boundaries; continuity of personnel;
continuity of information; and continuity over periods of time (including care out of hours). These themes are all pertinent to this book.

To many the topic of palliative care is still synonymous with cancer.
A diagnosis of cancer is becoming increasingly common in the UK
with one in three people being affected by the disease at some time
in their lives. Treatments such as chemotherapy and radiotherapy,
while increasingly successful, can be distressing and debilitating.
Patients and their carers are faced with life-threatening disease and
difficult treatment choices. They often need access to many different
services over time and may come across a large number of healthcare
professionals from different disciplines. Whilst the concept of 'living
with cancer' is becoming much more commonplace, with it comes
an expectation of survival, making the move from curative to palliative care a continuing difficult step for patients, their carers and the
health professionals involved.

This book is a welcome addition to the literature on palliative care.
It illuminates the importance of continuity of care and deals systematically with the subject. The editors have brought the relevant
knowledge about continuity in palliative care together into one text.
It provides practical information needed by primary care teams as
they care for what is likely to be an increasing number of patients

who will choose to die at home. Continuity of care issues are high-lighted across primary and secondary care, across hospital and hospice care, for patients and their carers with cancer and non-cancer palliative care, and for older people across health and social care.

This book provides a logical and ordered way of approaching the issues in the light of both new and well-established models of service delivery. Given the importance to the delivery of care of organisational boundaries, the relationship between continuity of care and cross-boundary issues facing primary care trusts is highlighted. In addition, the book offers thoughtful contributions on some wider aspects of palliative care, particularly communication, by including chapters on patient-held records and IT systems. Understanding the issues in palliative care that face primary care teams is an important concept in preparing for future challenges in the NHS and this book clearly, concisely and very readably summarises the story.

Professor Yvonne Carter  OBE MD FRCGP FMedSci
Dean, Warwick Medical School, University of Warwick
February 2007

# Authors

**Dr Dan Munday** MB BS DRCOG Dip Pall Med FFARCSI MRCGP is Consultant in Palliative Medicine for the Coventry PCT, Medical Director of Myton Hospice, Warwick, and Honorary Senior Clinical Lecturer at the Centre for Primary Health Care Studies, Warwick Medical School, University of Warwick. Trained in anaesthesia and general practice he worked as a GP principal for a number of years. Since 1998 he has worked in palliative medicine. His research interests are in community palliative care and its interface with primary care, research methodology and complexity theory. He is co-director of the Masters in Health Sciences (Palliative Care) at Warwick Medical School.

**Cathy Shipman** BA (Hons) MSc is Senior Research Fellow within both the Department of Palliative Care, Policy and Rehabilitation and the Department of General Practice and Primary Care at King's College, London. With a background in medical sociology she has worked principally in primary palliative care research for almost 10 years, and in primary health and social care research for most of her working life. Her research interests lie within primary palliative care and the work of district nurses, GPs, PCTs and specialist palliative care as well as the experiences and care of COPD and cancer patients.

**Professor Julia Addington-Hall** BA PhD HonMFPH is Professor of End of Life Care at the School of Nursing and Midwifery, Southampton University. She is a social scientist and leads the multidisciplinary Cancer, Palliative and End of Life Care Research Group at the School. Her research interests include the experiences of people who die from causes other than cancer, and in older age, methodological developments in palliative and end-of-life research, and mixed-method evaluations of health and social care services.

**Jenni Burt** BA (Hons) MSc is Research Fellow within the Department of Epidemiology and Public Health at University College London, and is currently supported by an MRC Special Training Fellowship in

Health Services Research. She has a degree in biological anthropology from Cambridge University and an MSc in public health from the London School of Hygiene and Tropical Medicine. In her current research, Jenni is investigating equity of use of specialist palliative care services; she also maintains an interest in the provision of palliative care within primary care, and the needs of vulnerable patient groups in the out-of-hours period.

**Dr Michael A. Cornbleet** BSc MD FRCP is Senior Medical Officer at the Scottish Executive Health Department. He trained in oncology in London and Edinburgh before being appointed as Consultant in Medical and Paediatric Oncology in Edinburgh in 1986. In 1993 he was appointed Medical Director at the Marie Curie Hospice in Edinburgh. Has a longstanding interest in developing research methods and capacity in palliative care.

**Dr Peter Ferry** MD MSc MRCP Dip Ger Dip ORT Cert Med Ed is Consultant Geriatrician at Zammit Clapp Hospital, Malta, Visiting Senior Clinical Lecturer in Medical Education at the University of Warwick and council member of the Malta Hospice Movement. His special interests include palliative care in older people, movement disorders and orthogeriatric rehabilitation.

**Dr Rob George** MA MD FRCP is Senior Lecturer in Bioethics and Philosophy of Medicine at University College London and Consultant in Palliative Medicine, Meadow House Hospice. He is a pioneer in developing services for those dying of HIV and in palliative care for patients with progressive disease of all diagnoses, establishing and leading the Palliative Care Centre at University College Hospital, London, for 17 years. In 2003 he moved to concentrate on research and teaching in bioethics at University College London, continuing his clinical practice as part of the team at Meadow House Hospice, West London.

**Dr J. Simon R. Gibbs** MB BChir MA MD FRCP is Senior Lecturer in Cardiology at Imperial College London and Honorary Consultant Cardiologist at Hammersmith Hospital. He is lead clinician for the National Pulmonary Hypertension service at Hammersmith and works in a multidisciplinary team consisting of junior doctors in training, specialist nurses, a health social worker and a chaplain. His research interests are in pulmonary hypertension, supportive and palliative care in cardiovascular disease, and high-altitude medicine. He is currently a member of the Circulatory and Respiratory Policy Group of the National Council for Palliative Care.

**Gloria Jones** DMS is Service Improvement Manager for Cancer and Palliative Care at Brent PCT. She has a background in management. Her commissioning experience has covered both primary and secondary care, including negotiation and performance monitoring. Through her involvement with the West London Cancer and Palliative Care Network, she has had a strategic role in the development of cancer and palliative care services in Brent PCT. She is very interested in equity in cancer/palliative care and access to relevant information for the diverse population of Brent.

**Dr Kashifa Mahmood** BA (Hons) MSc MPhil PhD is Research Fellow at the Centre for Primary Health Care Studies, Warwick Medical School, University of Warwick. Since May 2004 she has been Research Fellow for the Gold Standards Framework Evaluation Programme at Warwick. Previously she was a systematic reviewer for the development of NICE referral guidelines for suspected cancer. Since completing her doctorate at Manchester University in 2003 she has developed a research interest in cancer and health service policy and management.

**Professor Scott A. Murray** MD FRCP (Ed) FRCGP is St Columba's Professor of Primary Palliative Care, Division of Community Health Sciences, University of Edinburgh. He leads the Primary Palliative Care Research Group (www.chs.med.ed.ac.uk/gp/research/ppcrg. php), a multidisciplinary research team that seeks to understand the experiences of patients with life-limiting illnesses and their carers, and to develop and test best models of care. He has a vision for palliative care for all in need, irrespective of diagnosis or care setting.

**Canon Edward Pogmore** MA is Chaplaincy Coordinator for the George Eliot Hospital NHS Trust, Nuneaton, and the North

Warwickshire Primary Care NHS Trust. He has a Masters in health-care chaplaincy and is a non-residentiary canon of Coventry Cathedral. He leads the chaplaincy team in North Warwickshire and is Chairman of the Mary Ann Evans Hospice serving Northern Warwickshire and an external assessor in healthcare chaplaincy for the Department of Health.

**Angie Rogers** BA (Hons) MSc is Senior Research Fellow – End of Life Care at the School of Nursing and Midwifery, University of Southampton. She has worked in palliative care research for nearly 10 years and her research interests include care for non-cancer patients at the end of life, especially those with heart failure, stroke, CJD and dementia.

**Dr Wendy-Jane Walton** MB BS FRCGP is Part-Time Principal in General Practice in Shrewsbury and Macmillan End of Life Care Facilitator in Primary Care. She was awarded the RCGP 50th Anniversary Essay Prize 'Cum Scientia Caritas' in 2002, was the winner of the RSM John Fry Bursary in 2004, runner-up in 2005 and is a member of the Society of Medical Writers. Currently studying for the Diploma in Palliative Medicine at Cardiff University, she is married with three children and still has an awful lot of mountains left to climb.

**Dr Max Watson** BD MB BS MSc DRCOG DCH DMH MRCGP is Research Fellow in Palliative Medicine at Belfast City Hospital and Honorary Consultant at the Princess Alice Hospice, Esher. He has trained in general practice and palliative medicine, and his major research interests are anorexia and cachexia in patients with advanced disease, and in educating generalists in palliative care. He is the co-founder of the Certificate in Essential Palliative Care at Princess Alice Hospice and is author of *Oxford Handbook of Palliative Care* (Oxford University Press, 2005), *Oncology* (Oxford Core Texts) (Oxford University Press, 2006) and *Pain and Palliation* (Oxford University Press, 2007).

**Dr Allison Worth** BSc (Hons) PhD RGN RMN RHV is freelance researcher and Senior Research Fellow at the University of Edinburgh. She is a qualitative researcher with particular interests in palliative care for people with cancer and other long-term illnesses.

# Abbreviations

| | |
|---|---|
| **A&E** | accident and emergency |
| **CML** | chronic myeloid leukemia |
| **CNS** | clinical nurse specialist |
| **CoC** | continuity of care |
| **COPD** | chronic obstructive pulmonary disease |
| **CPVA** | Community Practitioners and Health Visitors Association |
| **DDS** | Doctors' Deputising Services |
| **DN** | district nurse |
| **DoH** | Department of Health |
| **EAU** | Emergency Admissions Unit |
| **ECN** | Emergency Care Network |
| **ECP** | Emergency Care Practitioners |
| **EoLCP** | End-of-Life Care Programme |
| **FHSAs** | Family Health Service Authorities |
| **GSF** | Gold Standards Framework |
| **HRG** | Healthcare Resource Group |
| **LCP** | Liverpool Care of the Dying Pathway |
| **LDP** | Local Delivery Plan |
| **MCA** | Mental Capacity Act 2005 |
| **NAGPC** | National Association of GP Cooperatives |
| **NCPC** | National Council for Palliative Care |
| **NICE** | National Institute for Health and Clinical Excellence |
| **NMC** | Nursing and Midwifery Council |
| **NSF** | National Service Framework |
| **NYHA** | New York Heart Association |
| **OOHDF** | Out of Hours Development Fund |
| **OT** | occupational therapist |
| **PALS** | Patient Advice and Liaison Service |
| **PBC** | Practice-Based Commissioning |
| **PCG** | Primary Care Group |
| **PCO** | Primary Care Organisation |
| **PCT** | Primary Care Trust |
| **PDA** | personal digital assistant |
| **PHR** | patient-held records |

**PPOC**  Preferred Place of Care
**QOF**  Quality and Outcomes Framework
**RCT**  randomised controlled trial
**SAP**  Single Assessment Process
**SDO**  NHS Service Delivery and Organisation Research and Development
**SLA**  Service Level Agreement
**SPC**  specialist palliative care
**SPCU**  Specialist Palliative Care Unit
**UCL**  University College London
**VOICES**  Views of Informal Carers – Evaluation of Services

CHAPTER | 1

# Introduction

Concepts, scope and models of continuity
in palliative care

*Dan Munday and Cathy Shipman*

The aim of this book is to look at the important areas involved in
achieving continuity in palliative care from the patient's, carer's
and professional health carer's perspective. This introductory chapter looks at some issues involved in the need for continuity of care,
exploring the various forms of continuity, highlighting some of the
obstacles to achieving continuity and suggesting a dynamic model
of continuity for palliative care. An outline of the chapters is given,
reflecting perspectives from primary, specialist and secondary care.
First, however, we focus on the changing circumstances of the palliative care patient and the importance of continuity of care.

## The palliative care patient and the importance of continuity

### Changing goals

For the patient with advanced non-curable cancer, the primary focus
of care should move from curative to the provision of supportive
and palliative care, with the aim of achieving the best quality of life.[1]
During the treatment phase of their disease the approach is to focus
primarily on the disease process, in order to achieve a cure, whilst
provision of supportive care is arguably of secondary importance.
In the palliative period particularly, which is when the disease is
advanced and cure is no longer feasible, supportive care becomes central and the management perspective needs to broaden, to focus on
the patient's wellbeing in terms of psychological, social and spiritual

needs in addition to treatment of physical symptoms. This change in the focus of care can be a difficult time for the patient, the patient's family and friends, and their healthcare professionals. Patients and their families not only have to cope with this change in approach to their healthcare management, but also they are often wrestling with existential questions resulting from their own, or their relative's, mortality.

Along with this change in management there often comes a change in the personnel intimately involved with the patient's care. For example, a patient may be discharged from the oncology clinic to be followed up more closely by a new set of professionals in the palliative care team. Ongoing input of their primary care team, particularly their general practitioner, can provide very important continuity at this time. Often they will have formed a relationship with their GP over many years, and the GP is likely to have shared their journey thus far from first presentation, diagnosis, treatment and remission to subsequent relapse. A district nurse (DN) may also become involved in patient care, perhaps making an introductory visit to establish the basis of a supportive relationship should nursing care be needed in the home as the disease progresses. From this point onwards until their inevitable death (and for their family into the grieving period) the need for continuity of care is paramount. Clearly identified roles for those professionals involved and good communication between professionals is vital to maintain such continuity of care.

For the patient with advanced non-malignant disease such as heart failure, the need for holistic palliative care is equally as great, but may not be so clearly recognised. Diagnosis of the terminal stage of disease may be more problematic[2] and management by specialist clinics may well need to continue into the palliative phase.[3] Many of these patients may not have access to specialist palliative care and other supportive care services, but continuity of care is vital since they face many similar problems to patients with advanced cancer.[4,5] These issues are developed to a greater extent in Chapter 8.

### Holistic care

Palliative care is necessarily holistic in its approach. In order for this to be achieved it is likely that many different healthcare professionals will need to bring their expertise to the patient's care. As is common with community health care in the United Kingdom, day-to-day provision of care falls to the primary care team: the general practitioner, district nurse, practice nurse, health visitor, surgery receptionist, practice-based counsellor and other professionals working within the primary care setting. The concept of holistic care has developed as a distinctive feature within the discipline of primary care[6,7] quite independently from its development within palliative care,[8] and is ideally extended to all patients – not just the palliative care patient.

Many skills needed for providing palliative care for patients with advanced disease are found within the primary care team, particularly within district nursing teams who often have extensive experience in this area. In addition, some primary care professionals have developed interests and skills over and above those considered to be core to the discipline. GPs may have developed a particular interest in symptom control of the palliative care patient, or psychological care, alternative therapies or in some other relevant medical speciality giving them particular expertise valuable in managing some palliative care patients. Many district nurses have developed a special interest in palliative care, having studied for diplomas or degrees in the area, in addition to possessing extensive knowledge and skills in the care of terminally ill patients from years of practice. Chapter 4 introduces issues of continuity of care important to the palliative care work of district nursing teams.

Many primary care teams, however, feel they need support from specialist palliative care services, particularly palliative care clinical nurse specialists (e.g. Macmillan nurses) and palliative medicine specialists[9] (see Chapter 6). Patients may attend hospice day care units that provide access to physiotherapy, counselling or alternative therapies. Day care attendance can help patients to maintain their independence within the community, to provide respite for their family carers and for specialist input for the control of troublesome, complex symptoms.[10] In addition patients may benefit from spiritual care from chaplains attached to the specialist palliative care team, often working closely with clergy or spiritual leaders from other faith groups within the community (see Chapter 9).

The need to involve many professionals in the patient's holistic care, particularly when it involves a variety of different healthcare teams, leads to the potential fragmentation of patient care. Poor communication amongst professionals – where individual practitioners do not have access to important information regarding decisions and the 'collusion of anonymity',[11] where no team member in the end takes responsibility for ensuring that care is delivered – are potential problems in palliative care. Unless these problems are appreciated, good communication between professionals is not seen as a high priority and there may be a system-related failure in providing high-quality care. Continuity of care is one of the first aspects of care to be lost when communication breaks down, potentially leading to loss of confidence of the patient and his or her family (see Chapter 5).

### Rapidly changing clinical situation

Patients with end-stage disease, particularly those with cancer, often have complex problems involving many different symptoms, some of which may be difficult to control. For instance, the majority of patients experience pain, many experiencing several 'types' of pain at the same time; many have other symptoms such as nausea and vomiting, constipation, breathlessness, cognitive impairment and psychological distress. In addition the patient's clinical state may change rapidly. This can make pre-planning care difficult and the situation may be compounded if new problems arise overnight or at a weekend, when their usual professional carers are not available. The need for emergency intervention by professionals unfamiliar with the patient's history can lead to unnecessary hospital admission, inappropriate management decisions and frustration on the part of the patient and their family. Regular follow-up by the primary care team therefore becomes necessary, with 'care planning' to anticipate problems as far as possible and information on the patient's care shared with colleagues covering out of hours, in an attempt to avoid this type of situation (see Chapters 2 and 11).

### Involving the whole family – communication problems

The patient needs to be seen within his or her social context. There are normally family and friends who are interested and concerned. Patients and their families want to know details of prognosis, likely course of the disease and problems that may be faced. They may be looking for reassurance and information regarding which services, if needed, might be available. This is all within the context of their struggle to come to terms with the illness and the shortening of life. Involving a multidisciplinary team in the care of the patient and family potentially leads to different and sometimes conflicting information being shared with them.

Part of the approach to this problem is to make sure that the whole team is skilled in communication, but also in ensuring that information is available to all staff involved with the patient. In addition, using one particular team member, who will normally be involved in sharing important pieces of information and helping the patient to interpret information being given to him or her, can be an important aspect in ensuring continuity of care.

### Current policies re 'access to care'

The need for palliative care patients to have access to appropriate care when it is needed has been highlighted by a number of recommendations from the government,[12-14] the National Institute for Health and Clinical Excellence (NICE)[15] and the specialist palliative care sector.[16] The problems faced by palliative care patients in out-of-hours periods were also highlighted in a report by Macmillan Cancer Relief[17] and Department of Health reports on out-of-hours care.[18] Attention to the provision of such care is an important aspect of palliative care strategy development by Primary Care Trusts (PCTs), specialist palliative care providers and cancer and palliative care networks. Palliative care is identified as an important element in National Service Frameworks (NSF)[19] for coronary heart disease, older people, long-term conditions and renal disease, highlighting the need for access to palliative care for patients with diseases other than cancer. Chapter 10 looks at the role of PCTs in terms of implementing government policy and organisational factors associated with barriers to the provision of continuity of care.

## Aspects of continuity of care

### *Theoretical aspects*

In planning for continuity of care, it is important to have a clear understanding of what is meant by continuity. From a review of academic and policy literature Haggerty and colleagues suggest that continuity of care comprises two distinct core elements, the care of an individual patient and care over time. They also distinguish three aspects of continuity:

- relational continuity – which is 'an ongoing therapeutic relationship between a patient and one or more carers'
- informational continuity – which involves the accessibility of information for individual patients
- managerial continuity – where the goals for patient care are shared and responsive to any changes in support and symptom control needs.[20]

Since patients at the end of life often experience repeated admissions to hospital or hospice, we would add a fourth aspect to the three defined by Haggerty *et al.*, that of continuity of place as developed by Rogers *et al.* in Chapter 8. The place in which a patient finds himself or herself will be related to his or her proposed or actual management, and relational continuity will also be contingent on place. Relational, managerial and continuity of place are the aspects of which patients are most aware. Conversely, whilst patients will not normally be aware of informational continuity, it may become apparent to them in situations where it is lacking, for example when they need to repeat their history to unfamiliar professionals (see Chapter 5). Relational, managerial and informational continuity and continuity of place should be maintained to enable effective care to be delivered over time. These may therefore be considered as *longitudinal aspects* of continuity (see Figure 1.1).

Freeman *et al.* propose that continuity needs to be maintained within and between teams as well as between practitioners.[21] This is particularly relevant for palliative care patients, because care for them is often delivered *simultaneously* by several multidisciplinary teams (from primary, secondary and occasionally tertiary care). These aspects can therefore be considered as *cross-sectional* continuity.

Figure 1.1 **Longitudinal continuity of care**

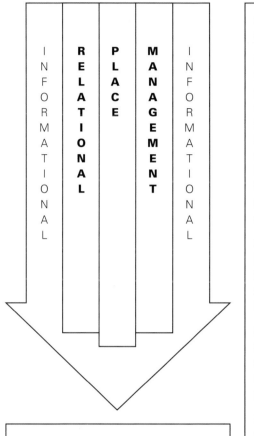

INFORMATIONAL | RELATIONAL | PLACE | MANAGEMENT | INFORMATIONAL

**'Arrow of time'**

The patient *experiences* continuity of *relationship* and *management*. Information is necessary to ensure this continuity

**Aspects of longitudinal continuity**

*Relational* – care received from a single professional or group of professionals. *Personal continuity*, e.g. from a single general practitioner, Macmillan nurse counsellor, chaplain, etc. This may be formalised with a named key worker. *Team continuity*, e.g. district nurse team, oncology team

*Place* – e.g. home, hospital, hospice, nursing /residential home. Will be affected by *management* and will have an impact on *relational continuity*

*Management* – holistic care (physical, psychological, social and spiritual): coherent with common aims, integrated and coordinated

*Informational* – enables management and relational continuity. *Information* – notes, letters, etc. *Knowledge of the patient* – retained by practitioner/team through personal or shared knowledge

For example, a patient may be receiving palliative radiotherapy from the oncology team, symptom control advice from the palliative care team, syringe driver management from the district nursing team and psychological support from a counsellor (see Figure 1.2a).

This book is not concerned with palliative care for cancer patients

Figure 1.2a **Cross-sectional continuity – a model of care for cancer**

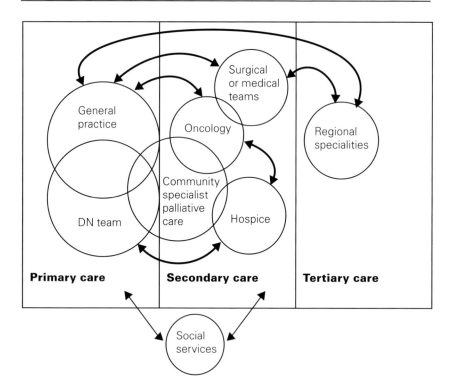

*Note*: the patient may experience care delivered from several (occasionally all) of these services at any one time. Through time the relative involvement of each will vary.

*Key: overlapping circles* represent teams that have direct contact with each other, while arrows represent communication without direct contact, e.g. by letter, fax, etc.

alone, and Figure 1.2b suggests a model of care for a patient dying from heart failure.

These aspects of continuity arise explicitly and implicitly throughout this book. We will therefore discuss them in some detail in the following sections before returning to develop a model of continuity for palliative care.

## Relational continuity

Relational continuity includes both personal continuity of care with a single practitioner and care provided by a team. Patients

Figure 1.2b **Cross-sectional continuity – a model of care for heart failure**

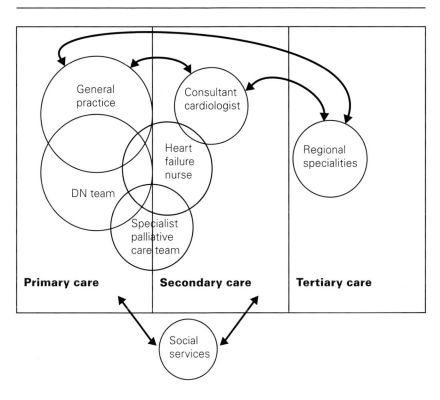

*Note*: the patient may experience care delivered from several (occasionally all) of these services at any one time. Through time the relative involvement of each will vary.

*Key: overlapping circles* represent teams that have direct contact with each other, while arrows represent communication without direct contact, e.g. by letter, fax, etc.

with advanced cancer will often see large numbers of doctors in their progress through the hospital system. One study showed that patients with advanced cancer saw on average 28 doctors during the first year from diagnosis.[22] Personal continuity therefore has much to recommend it in the management of the palliative care patient as it encourages the development of a trusting relationship and consistent communication. However, it can lead to a lack of multidisciplinary input, unless the practitioner providing the personal continuity is prepared to share care with other team members. Total continuity given by one person is also almost never feasible since the practitioner would need to be available continuously.

### Historical aspects

At the time of the inception of the NHS in the UK, the GP would provide personal continuity of care for his or her patients.[23] All UK residents have until recently been entitled to be registered with a single general practitioner, who is contracted to provide 24-hour care, 365 days per year. Following the implementation of the new GP contract in 2004, registration is now with the practice rather than the individual GP. The contractual changes may not affect the public perception of having a personal GP, since most GPs work in group practices and many patients in any case would have seen *their doctor* as being different from the GP with whom they were actually registered. In the early decades of the NHS, GPs provided care for their patient's acute and chronic illness both in the surgery and the patient's home. GPs would also be responsible for antenatal care and obstetric interventions. Whilst a GP may have managed patients in the immediate post-myocardial infarct stage at home, the general rule was that general medical specialists managed medical conditions, such as hypertension, diabetes and asthma, in hospital outpatient clinics.[23]

As a result of the increasing technological advances in medical practice and changes within health care and wider society, the GP's role has changed dramatically. Childbirth rarely now occurs at home under the care of the GP. Patients do not stay at home following a myocardial infarction as in the past. However, treatment of diabetes, hypertension and asthma, and performance of minor surgical procedures, are now a part of GP provision with many GPs receiving special training in these areas. The GP not only provides care for the unwell but is also expected to provide health promotion advice, preventative health care such as vaccination programmes and screening for potential early or pre-clinical disease in the healthy.

Fewer home visits are performed in general, partly because patients are more mobile but also because home visits are an inefficient way to provide a service. GPs more commonly work in partnerships, with patients often seeing different GPs according to availability or preference. The emphasis has also moved from general practice to 'primary care', and the delivery of primary care is now focused on a multidisciplinary team rather than on the individual GP. GPs are still largely responsible for the 'gate-keeping' role on the primary–secondary care interface, though no longer exclusively so, especially with the development of specialist nurse and nurse practitioner roles. Access to care is likely to change further as part of imminent and potentially radical changes to the provision of care outside hospitals, as discussed in more depth in the final chapter.

Many GPs are still drawn towards caring for the palliative care patient, since they identify that, in this area, personal continuity of care and the traditional role of GP or family doctor remains of value.[24] Few GPs are able to offer 24-hour personal continuity of care due to other demands on their time with the extended role of primary care and changes in out-of-hours practice. Some GPs, however, will still give the family their personal telephone number within a few days of the patient's death. These issues are developed in greater depth in Chapter 2.

### New models of personal or relational continuity of care

Although the model of GPs providing continuous personal care is largely historical, other aspects of personal continuity of care remain. Many GPs still visit palliative care patients regularly and take a personal interest in the patient's ongoing care within the setting of the multidisciplinary team.[25] Often, however, it is the DN who provides personal continuity of care, visiting increasingly frequently towards the very end of life. The GP may often leave this aspect of care to them, in recognition of their expertise in palliative care and partly because of lack of time for such activities. Since DNs work in teams, relational continuity might be offered by a team of two or three nurses rather than a single district nurse. Relational continuity with the district nursing team is often highly valued (see Chapter 5).

In some areas of health care, notably mental health, the concept of a key worker has developed in which one member of the team is given particular responsibility for providing personal continuity to patients.[26] This has perhaps been less common in palliative care although it has now been formalised through the Gold Standards Framework for Palliative Care (see Chapter 11) and through the NICE *Guidance on Cancer Services: Improving supportive and palliative care for adults*.[15] Whilst a formalised key worker role has been uncommon in palliative care, unwritten contracts have perhaps more commonly appeared between a patient and a professional carer to fulfil this role.

The advantage of this informal approach is that it allows the patient to exercise choice in who they see as their 'key worker', but the main drawback is that it may lead to unsustainable pressures on the health-care workers and overdependence on an individual practitioner by patients and their families. These issues are developed to a greater extent in Chapter 7 concerning continuity of care for the elderly and Chapter 8 for those suffering from non-malignant disease.

It remains to be seen how the practice of personal continuity of care will develop and who will offer this in palliative care following recent changes within the NHS, not least within the GP contract (see Chapter 10 and 15).

**Managerial continuity of care**

Care for the palliative patient needs to be individually tailored since all patients will have a unique set of problems needing to be addressed. Physical, psychological, social and spiritual problems should be addressed simultaneously, with management discussed and agreed with the patient and carers. Management is therefore complex, often involving several professionals from different teams with changing clinical needs requiring frequent adjustment of management plans. This can lead to a bewildering experience for the patient, even when management is logical and ordered from the perspective of healthcare professionals. Poor attention to detail, lack of communication and unavailability of information all mitigate against coherent and integrated care. In order to ensure managerial continuity, effective communication of information between professionals and teams needs to be achieved.

**Continuity within teams**

Continuity of care by the primary and palliative care multidisciplinary team should be ensured at all times with shared goals for patient care and support. The patient's care should be discussed at multidisciplinary team meetings, when a clear decision as to which professional to be involved in any given situation should be made. Decisions should be clearly recorded for reference at a later date and for clinical governance purposes.

At times concern is expressed regarding the loss of patient confidentiality in these circumstances. This can be avoided by explaining to the patient the nature of the multidisciplinary team and sharing information on a 'need to know' basis. Patient information should always be treated as confidential to the team and all practitioners are bound by their professional codes of confidentiality (see Chapter 14). When a member of the team involved with a patient's care is absent, a deputy should be appointed to ensure continuity if the patient requires input whilst the usual team member is absent.

### Continuity across primary, secondary and tertiary care

Palliative care patients may be under the care of teams from primary, secondary (i.e. locally based specialist) and tertiary (i.e. regional or national specialist) care. This is especially so for patients with rare tumour or disease types, or those receiving experimental treatment. Shared goals for patient care should be agreed with the patient, with an understanding of those goals shared between teams. Therefore, communication and collaboration between teams is vital to enable such shared understanding of goals. Unfortunately this is one of the aspects of continuity that not uncommonly fails. It is often extremely difficult for members of primary care teams to attend secondary care-convened multidisciplinary meetings and vice versa, but communication should be maintained by regular correspondence, telephone communication and joint visiting whenever feasible, e.g. DN/GP and specialist joint visits. Continuity is more likely to be maintained if the teams cover the same geographical area and are coterminous with each other, since knowledge of local working practices by other teams and personal relationships develop as teams work closely together.

Problems arise more commonly when teams are from different localities and are not familiar with each other's practices. On the borders between services a patient may receive care from a primary care team in one PCT area, but a specialist team from another. When social service delivery is also taken into account these problems may be compounded. In addition, specialist palliative care may be delivered by more than one provider in a given area partly as a result of the development of individual hospice services within the voluntary sector and with some aspects of care provided by independent pro-viders and some by NHS providers (see Chapter 6).

Similar problems occur when palliative care teams work across the boundaries of more than one cancer centre. Problems of coordina-tion of cross-boundary care are being currently addressed by cancer and palliative care networks.[27] In some areas the situation can be extremely complex. For instance, in one area of the West Midlands the local specialist palliative care team work across five separate cancer networks, necessitating the development of systems for continuity across all of these networks.

When multiple teams from different levels of care are involved, the problems of communication are compounded. Rapid communication between primary, secondary and tertiary care may in the future be achieved by the development of the NHS IT strategy and the 'single patient record'. It remains to be seen whether this is an achievable objective and what problems such a system will develop (see the next section).

Continuity of care across sectors can be particularly problematic for some vulnerable groups of patients, for example the elderly, who often suffer co-morbidities and may have difficulty in accessing spe-cialist palliative care and other services, as explored in Chapter 7. Lack of access to specialist palliative care services is also common to many people suffering from progressive non-malignant disease, and continuity of care between primary and secondary sectors may be compromised by acute exacerbations and the need for urgent hospi-tal admission (see Chapter 8).

## Continuity of information

All healthcare professionals should have access to information that is up to date in order to manage the palliative care patient appropriately and effectively. Many different professionals within several different teams may see individual palliative care patients. Often, each one of these different professionals keeps separate case notes. For instance, it is not uncommon for a patient to have separate notes regarding their present illness being kept by the GP, district nursing service, specialist palliative care nurse, in-patient hospice, day care hospice, local general hospital, clinical oncologist in the sub-regional cancer centre and tertiary specialist in a regional centre. Results of tests may not be available in all sets of records, e.g. blood test results may have been made available to the oncologist, surgeon and GP but not the palliative team. Incomplete sets of letters regarding the patient may be filed in each of the sets of notes, no professional having a complete set.

The option to have one set of combined notes is not feasible if care is given by different institutions. Secondary care for cancer is not only provided by oncology and palliative care specialists but also by hospital generalists, who may well have their own systems for keeping and storing notes that may not be compatible with the needs of the cancer specialist teams. If unified notes are kept, time is taken in transporting them and there is the potential that they will be 'lost in the system' or needed almost simultaneously in more than one site.

Storing notes on a central computer server potentially overcomes this problem since such notes can be accessed electronically at all connected sites. This, however, will require many different institutions, both independent and NHS, to operate compatible systems, which raises major resource and organisational issues. The NHS is now addressing these issues with the £6bn 'National Programme for IT' (NPfIT).[28] The project has not been without controversy (including the escalation of costs) and the clinical utility of such a project for a complex area such as palliative care remains unknown. In addition, moving to the electronic record also requires staff, with varying degrees of computer literacy, to learn new ways of note keeping. Some aspects of record keeping, for example recording narrative or diagrams, are more difficult to achieve on electronic systems. Therefore the introduction of the electronic record normally leads to the time-consuming problem of double data entry, which will remain until the total electronic record becomes feasible (see Chapter 13).

Patient-held records provide another way of enabling continuity of information but require the commitment of all professionals involved to make sure that the notes are kept up to date (see Chapter 12). The practice of leaving district nursing notes within the patient's home does provide a useful if incomplete method of recording information for other professionals in the situation where the patient is housebound and is receiving regular district nurse input.

Continuity of information is important, especially when there is little continuity of personal care, such as in the out-of-hours setting. Primary care teams should be encouraged to pass on important information to their 'on call colleagues', although this information will necessarily be incomplete and can become rapidly out of date. (This is discussed in Chapter 2.)

In addition to information recorded in case notes (paper and electronic), clinical letters or handover sheets, information is also retained about the patient by individual practitioners. This information could be described as *knowledge of the patient*, and is reliant on relational continuity. Such knowledge is difficult to record for others to access and its importance may be overlooked in systems designed to provide clinical information.

**Continuity of place of care**

The majority of patients express a wish to be cared for in their own homes. Continuity of place of care is only possible where sufficient support and resources can be provided for both patients and carers. Palliative care patients have high levels of need, sometimes requiring complex therapeutic interventions including symptom control and/or nursing care. Admission to hospital or hospice can become necessary even with the availability of enhanced community services whose aim is to allow patients to remain at home. Movement between different care contexts clearly represents a break in continuity. Careful planning involving all relevant health professionals and including the patient and carers should facilitate coherent and integrated care, and will enable breaks in continuity of place to be as smooth as possible. Unfortunately, examples given in Chapter 5 on patient and carer experiences with out-of-hours and emergency care show that this is not always achieved.

Supporting patients and carers to enable patients to remain at home for as long as possible, and to die at home where this is preferred, is the focus of the government's end-of-life care strategy and earlier policies.[13,14] This strategy and the programmes designed to facilitate its implementation are described in detail in Chapter 11.

## A model for continuity of palliative care

As has already been discussed, continuity can be considered in terms of continuity over time (longitudinal continuity) and continuity between individual practitioners and teams (cross-sectional continuity) (Figures 1.1, 1.2a and 1.2b). We would propose that this forms the basis of a useful model for continuity in palliative care. It is important to stress, however, that continuity in palliative care is a *dynamic* rather than a *static* process. The representation of cross-sectional continuity (Figures 1.2a and 1.2b) will change over time, since, as new professionals or teams become involved, others will become less prominent or cease involvement with patient care altogether, e.g. when a patient is discharged from a surgical or oncology clinic.

A useful conceptual framework for this dynamic approach is provided by complexity theory,[29] which proposes that complex systems – of which the patient, the patient's social networks and health professional teams caring for the patient are examples – co-evolve over time in a largely unpredictable though not a random manner. The interactions between the various elements of the system have a crucial effect on how the system evolves. The system can be relatively stable for long periods, followed by rapid change even as a result of small events or interactions between elements. Attempts to predict outcomes for the patient are therefore problematic and the emergent course of care may vary markedly in different situations. A worked example to illustrate this is given in Box 1.1.

## Obstacles to continuity

Many obstacles to continuity have already been discussed. Finally, however, we will concentrate on three important areas where problems can particularly arise. Within these three areas lie threats to the core components of continuity of care.

### Out of hours

Achieving continuity of care during the out-of-hours period (i.e. evenings, nights, weekends and public holidays) can be problematic.[30] Many within palliative care reacted negatively to the formation of GP cooperatives, although the evidence has not been convincing that

---

Box 1.1 **Worked example of the emergent course of care**

---

Three months ago, Ted Jones, a 67-year-old retired lorry driver living at home with his daughter and her family, was diagnosed with lung cancer at an advanced stage. He has undergone palliative chemotherapy and radiotherapy, ending one month ago. Despite this he has been gradually deteriorating. He has expressed a wish to die at home.

He has a syringe driver with drugs for pain and nausea that was started during an admission to a local hospice with vomiting and poor pain control. He is under the care of a consultant clinical oncologist, community palliative care clinical nurse specialist (CNS) and district nurses (DN) who change his syringe driver daily. His GP, who has known him and his family for 20 years, also visits every other week and regularly discusses management with the DN and CNS at a practice team meeting and at other times as necessary. Management information is kept up to date in the district nursing record in the home, and a fax detailing important aspects of history and management has been sent to the out-of-hours provider following the hospice discharge when the last significant management change was made.

One Friday afternoon he becomes short of breath; both the GP and DN are called but are unavailable as they are in an education session on palliative care. The daughter calls the CNS who makes an emergency visit, finding him quite distressed, with noisy breathing, and the daughter frightened. The CNS, deciding she needs further advice, speaks to the clinical oncologist responsible for his care. Mr Jones is admitted to hospital where he is found to have a chest infection. Despite treatment with antibiotics he deteriorates and dies in hospital.

*Notes*: this case illustrates exemplary practice in terms of multidisciplinary teamworking and communication, leading to relational and management continuity and continuity of place. However, in the end the patient does not achieve his wish to die at home. The factors are an unforeseen problem and unavailability of the GP (disruption of personal continuity) reinforced by increasing anxiety in the patient, daughter and CNS. If the GP had been present he might have diagnosed a chest infection, and, because he knew the patient and family well (*knowledge of patient*), along with his expertise as a GP, calmed the situation and treated the patient at home (*continuity of place*). As it was, the CNS, unable to make a diagnosis and less familiar with the patient and family, was not in a position to reassure; she took appropriate action in speaking to the clinical oncologist, who knew the patient although not the family, and was not able to make a home assessment. The patient was therefore admitted to hospital.

care given since the formation of cooperatives in the last 10 years has worsened. Recent changes to out-of-hours provision as a result of the new GP contract are still too new to evaluate. However, since the majority of GPs have opted out of being responsible for the delivery of primary care for their patients out of hours, the impact on delivery of palliative care may be much greater than that occurring with the development of cooperatives. Wendy-Jane Walton's personal view (Chapter 3), describing experiences working in a GP out-of-hours cooperative, provides a useful insight into how continuity for palliative care patients may be maintained through a GP's effective use of clinical and communication skills.

Community nursing services, providing both qualified district nursing and 'night sitting' for seriously ill patients remaining at home, are acknowledged as being necessary for continuity of palliative care out of hours.[31] These services are known to be 'patchy' with some patients being denied a comprehensive service.[32] Community nurses will often feel unsupported by lack of specialist services (e.g. Macmillan nurses), which is often a feature of these out-of-hours periods. In addition, working with on-call GPs with whom they are unfamiliar may also be problematic, and mistrust and misunderstandings can easily arise. The lack of equity regarding access to out-of-hours services can be seen as an example of 'postcode provision' and is a major area of concern.

### *Professional practices and perceptions*

Provision of holistic care for palliative care patients with rapidly changing complex needs and for their families is best provided through the development of personalised care plans by multidisciplinary teams. For these teams to function effectively there needs to be a clear understanding of the role that each member plays and respect for their professional knowledge, skills and practices. This process will require individual team members to be prepared to acknowledge differences in perspective brought by professionals from other disciplines, to be prepared to find team consensus and sometimes to allow their own views not to be followed. Poor understanding of each other's perspectives, especially between medical and nursing staff and between primary and secondary palliative care can lead to tensions within the team and fragmented and substandard care.[33] Repeated conflict within a team leads to dysfunctional relationships, rivalry and ultimately the destruction of the team. Occasionally patients can become aware of professional differences due to inadvisable comments by individual professionals that can lead to confusion and anger. Ultimately decisions need to be taken that all team members may not agree upon. In these situations clear but sensitive leadership and respect for decisions by all team members is vital. This is explored further in Chapter 14.

Local agreements on provision of care, communication and referral procedures should be sought and acted upon. Individual practitioners and professional groupings should be free to express their opinions and concerns in a climate of openness. Joint initiatives for audit and clinical governance will help to foster such a climate of mutual respect and support.[34]

### The paradox of patient choice

A key concept of continuity of care is *individualised care* provided to patients and carers. Patient choice as well as equity of access to appropriate services is an important feature within the new NHS.[13,14] An emphasis on patient autonomy and changes in expectations within society have largely driven the move for patients to be able to choose the most appropriate care for them. This is in contrast to the previous rather paternalistic expectation that the public would accept that 'doctor or nurse knows best' and therefore receive the treatment being offered without question. It is now accepted that patients have a right to full information about services that are available and are thus able to make informed choices as to the care they receive. Increased choice, however, has to be balanced against the resource implications of providing a large variety of services. At times when services are unavoidably restricted, e.g. in the out-of-hours period, patient choice is likely to continue to be limited.

A further difficulty that emerges through being presented with a wide variety of options is knowing which service to choose at what time. Salisbury has pointed out that patients in the out-of-hours period are faced with a potentially bewildering decision about who to call. Should it be their GP or out-of-hours GP provider, the district nurse or NHS Direct? Should they call for an ambulance or go to the accident and emergency department, the walk-in centre or the local primary care 'on call' centre.[35] Palliative care patients may also have the option of calling the local hospice or 'on call' palliative care nurse specialist.

Making a decision as to who to call is likely to be affected by numerous factors. These include previous experience, the relationship they have with a particular professional or service, the service that they feel is most appropriate and likely to be available, and the advice of friends and relatives, in addition to the information that they have been given by professional carers (see Chapter 5).

## Conclusion

Providing continuity of care in an increasingly complex and technological health service is a challenge and is likely to continue to be problematic. It is not possible to turn the clock back to a period when patients received personal continuity of care from the traditional 'family doctor'. Some have even suggested that this never really existed and is a myth that has grown up as a result of rapid change and uncertainty within the health service.[36] However, we believe there is scope to provide equitable, high-quality services with continuity of care and patient choice as important principles. For these services to function effectively they need to be properly planned, resourced and evaluated. We aim in this book to present some of the important issues, results of research and examples of good practice.

## REFERENCES

1. *Cancer Pain Relief and Palliative Care: Technical Report Series 804.* Geneva: World Health Organization, 1990.

2. Murray S, Kendall M, Boyd K and Sheikh A. Illness trajectories and palliative care. *British Medical Journal* 2005; **330**: 1007–11.

3. Gibbs J S R, McCoy A S M, Gibbs L, Rogers A E and Addington-Hall J M. Living with and dying from heart failure: The role of palliative care. *Heart* 2002; **88 (suppl. 11)**: ii 36–ii 39.

4. Addington-Hall J, Fakhoury W and McCarthy M. Specialist palliative care in nonmalignant disease. *Palliative Medicine* 1998; **12 (6)**: 417–27.

5. Murray S, Boyd K and Sheikh A. Palliative care in chronic illness. *British Medical Journal* 2005; **330**: 611–12.

6. McWhinney I. Primary care: Core values. Core values in a changing world. *British Medical Journal* 1998; **316**: 1807–9.

7. Heath I and Sweeney K. Medical generalists: Connecting the map and the territory. *British Medical Journal* 2005; **331 (7530)**: 1462–4.

8. Fordham S, Dowrick C and May C. Palliative medicine: Is it really specialist territory. *Journal of the Royal Society of Medicine* 1998; **91**: 568–72.

9. Barclay S, Todd C, McCabe J and Hunt T. Primary care group commissioning of services: The differing priorities of general practitioners and district nurses for palliative care services. *British Journal of General Practice* 1999; **49**: 181–6.

10. Higginson IJ, Hearn J, Myers K and Naysmith A. Palliative day care: What do services do? Palliative Day Care Project Group. *Palliative Medicine* 2000; **14 (4)**: 277–86.

11. Balint M. *The Doctor, His Patient and the Illness.* London: Churchill Livingstone, 2000.

12. E L (96) 85 *A Policy Framework for Commissioning Cancer Services: Palliative care services.* London: NHS Executive, 1996.

13. *The NHS Cancer Plan: A plan for investment, a plan for reform.* London: Department of Health, 2000.

14. *Building on the Best: Choice, responsiveness and equity in the NHS.* London: Department of Health, 2003.

15. *Guidance on Cancer Services: Improving supportive and palliative care for adults.* London: National Institute for Clinical Excellence, 2004.

16. Tebbit P. *Palliative Care 2000: Commissioning through partnership.* London: National Council for Hospices and Specialist Palliative Care, 1999.

17. Thomas K. *Out of Hours Palliative Care in the Community.* London: Macmillan Cancer Relief, 2001.

18. *Raising Standards for Patients: New partnerships in out of hours care.* London: Department of Health, 2000.

19. National Service Frameworks [web page]. Available at: www.dh.gov.uk/
    PolicyAndGuidance/HealthAndSocialCareTopics/HealthAndSocialCare
    Article/fs/en?CONTENT_ID=4070951&chk=W3ar/W [accessed March 2007].

20. Haggerty J, Reid R, Freeman G, Starfield B, Adair C and McKendry R. Continuity
    of care: A multidisciplinary review. *British Medical Journal* 2003; **327**: 1219–21.

21. Freeman G, Shephard S, Robertson I, Ehrich K and Richards S. *Continuity of Care:
    Report of a scoping exercise.* London: National Health Service, Service Delivery and
    Organisation, National Research and Development Programme, 2000.

22. Smith S, Nicol K, Devereux J and Cornbleet M. Encounters with doctors: Quantity
    and quality. *Palliative Medicine* 1999; **13**: 217–23.

23. Berger J M J. *A Fortunate Man.* London: RCGP, 2003.

24. Field D. Special not different: General practitioners' accounts of their care of dying
    people. *Social Science and Medicine* 1998; **46 (9)**: 1111–20.

25. Jeffrey D. *Cancer: From cure to care.* Manchester: Hochland & Hochland, 2000.

26. Tyrer P, Morgan J, Van Horn E, *et al.* A randomised controlled study of close
    monitoring of vulnerable psychiatric patients. *Lancet* 1995; **345 (8952)**: 756–9.

27. *The NHS Cancer Plan: A plan for investment, a plan for reform.* London: Department
    of Health, 2000.

28. *Connecting for Health: National programme for IT in the NHS* [web page]. Available at:
    www.connectingforhealth.nhs.uk/ [accessed March 2007].

29. Munday D, Johnson S and Griffiths F. Complexity theory and palliative care.
    *Palliative Medicine* 2003; **17**: 308–9.

30. Thomas K. Out of hours palliative care – bridging the gap. *European Journal of
    Palliative Care* 2000; **7 (1)**: 22–5.

31. Thorpe G. Enabling more dying people to remain at home. *British Medical Journal*
    1993; **307**: 915–18.

32. Munday D, Dale J and Barnett M. Out of hours palliative care in the UK:
    Perspectives from general practice and specialist services. *Journal of the Royal Society
    of Medicine* 2002; **95**: 28–30.

33. Seymour J, Clark D, Hughes P, *et al.* Clinical nurse specialists in palliative care.
    Part 3. Issues for the Macmillan nurse role. *Palliative Medicine* 2002; **16**: 386–94.

34. Munday D. Clinical governance and palliative care. In: Charlton R, ed. *Primary
    Palliative Care.* Oxford: Radcliffe Medical Press, 2002, pp. 15–29.

35. Salisbury C. Out of hours care: Ensuring accessible high quality care for all groups
    of patients. *British Journal of General Practice* 2000; **50 (455)**: 443–4.

36. Mihill C. *Shaping Tomorrow: Issues facing general practice in the new millennium.*
    London: British Medical Association, 2000.

CHAPTER | 2

# General practice and out-of-hours palliative care

*Dan Munday and Cathy Shipman*

## Introduction

General practice in the UK has been the bedrock of the National Health Service since its inception nearly 60 years ago. People resident in the UK have been able to access health care that is 'free at the point of need' at the time when they need it, through their local general practitioner. Until very recently everybody has been entitled to be registered with a GP, who has been contracted by their local Primary Care Organisation (PCO), to provide 24-hour 'general medical services'. Since the new GP contract was adopted in 2004, patients are now registered with a practice, rather than an individual GP, and practices can opt out of providing 24-hour care.

Not only have GPs been the 'gate-keepers' to the rest of the health service, but they have also been seen as experts in the provision of health care within the family and wider social context, such that 'the general practitioner engages with autonomous individuals across the fields of prevention, diagnosis, cure, care, and palliation, using and integrating the sciences of biomedicine, medical psychology, and medical sociology'.[1] Personal continuity of care is also seen as being a central feature of general practice. Although evidence that this is essential in providing effective care is lacking[2] it is an aspect highly valued by patients[3] and GPs themselves.[4] Vulnerable patients, such as those with terminal illness, are also likely to highly value continuity, as do GPs in caring for these patients.[5,6]

The practice of GPs in providing out-of-hours care for palliative care patients has, since 1995, come under great scrutiny, for arguably three reasons. Firstly, it was in 1995 that the provision of out-of-hours care in general practice changed radically and rapidly, with new regulations governing out-of-hours remuneration. In addition an out-of-hours development fund, which enabled GPs to set up coopera-tives (non-profit-making organisations of 10 or more GP principals), providing out-of-hours care for patients of members was established.[7] Secondly, several research studies at this time presented evidence that many carers were not always highly satisfied with care received from GPs[8] and highlighted potential deficiencies in palliative care training[9] and symptom control practices by GPs.[10] Finally, the estab-lishment of the Macmillan GP palliative care facilitator programme, a group of GP champions for palliative care in the primary care setting, provided a focus for the examination and development of GP practices in palliative care, including out-of-hours provision.[11]

The aim of this chapter is to examine the changes in out-of-hours general practice in the past 10 years and to examine the issues surrounding the care of palliative care patients, both from the perspective of research evidence and examples of good practice. The recent implementation of a new GP contract[12] will have argu-ably more far-reaching implications for the provision of out-of-hours palliative care in the community than any of the preceding changes described. However, much has been learned through research and experience, and it is vital that any new service design takes account of this evidence.

## Summary of GP out-of-hours services before 1995

Patients have had the choice to access health care through attendance at an accident and emergency department (A&E) or by calling the ambulance service. However, the normal route, except in an extreme emergency or as a result of an acute injury, has been through their registered GP. At the beginning of the 1990s, it became apparent that GPs' workload out of hours had gradually increased[13] over the pre-vious 30 years.[14] The way GPs organised out-of-hours care had also changed, with few GPs offering personal services out of hours. At that time it was estimated that two-thirds of GPs worked in practice rotas for some or all of their out-of-hours cover, with 30 per cent using collaboration with neighbouring practices.[14] Also, this period saw the rise in out-of-hours primary care being provided by deputising services – commercial organisations that GPs contracted to provide services for their patients. Doctors Deputising Services (DDS) were at this time available for GPs in most city and larger urban areas. Between 1977 and 1989 it was estimated that around 40 per cent of GPs used deputising services at least some of the time.[14]

Reasons for the increased demand for out-of-hours care are complex and remain largely speculative.[15] An important factor, however, was arguably a rise in consumerism in society and in the demand for health care. Such societal changes would not only have increased patient demand for health care at a time and place of their choosing, but also affected GPs' willingness to provide 24-hour care at the expense of their own personal life.[4] When surveyed in 1992, 57 per cent of general practitioners believed that 24-hour responsibility was outdated, 82 per cent agreed that it should be possible to opt out of providing 24-hour care and 73 per cent said that they would like to do so.[16]

As a result of the general dissatisfaction amongst GPs new rules were negotiated in 1995 whereby GPs would not be penalised for working in large rotas (since 1990 GPs had only attracted a higher night visit fee if they worked in a rota of 10 or fewer doctors). The government also announced a £45 million out-of-hours development fund principally to allow GPs to set up cooperative arrangements for providing out-of-hours services.[17]

## 1995 onwards – the rise of the GP out-of-hours cooperative

A GP cooperative is defined as 'a non profit making organisation entirely and equally owned by and mostly medically staffed by the GP principals of the area in which it operates'.[18] The first cooperatives had been set up in the 1970s, mainly as a result of local agreement with Family Health Service Authorities (FHSAs), which were at that time responsible for contracting health services with GPs. It was not until the changes in payment rules and the setting up of the Out of Hours Development Fund that cooperatives became viable to the majority of GPs. After 1995 cooperative numbers increased rapidly, so that by 1998 there were 22,000 GP members of cooperatives throughout the UK.[19] This represented the GPs responsible for between 70 per cent and 80 per cent of the UK population.

Cooperatives varied in many aspects including: size – from 10 to 400 GP members, covering 12,000 to over 1 million registered patients; area covered – urban/suburban, rural or mixed; management structure – loosely knit 'clubs' to limited companies with a management board and AGM of GP members. Other variations included employment of staff – telephonists, drivers, triage nurses; GP rota arrangements – equally shared rotas amongst members, employment of some GPs to do specific shifts, or subcontracting with DDS to cover home visiting.[19] It is therefore impossible to generalise or compare the activities of cooperatives apart from in descriptive terms.

The majority of cooperatives became members of the National Association of GP Cooperatives (NAGPC), which had the stated aim of representing and supporting member cooperatives and in promoting quality in out-of-hours care. Through a series of conferences and regular newsletters and 'information faxes' the member cooperatives were kept in touch with important issues in out-of-hours general practice and primary care, and were able to share good practice. The NAGPC identified many benefits of belonging to a cooperative (see Box 2.1).

**Satisfaction with out-of-hours arrangements and outcomes of care**

Early studies of GPs belonging to cooperatives showed high levels of satisfaction with both their personal benefits and standards of patient care.[20,21] Patients interestingly showed equal levels of satisfaction with all GP out-of-hours arrangements, but were largely unsatisfied with telephone consultations, when their expectations were not met in terms of how their call was dealt with [23-5] and with delays in visiting.[25,26] A randomised controlled trial, comparing a practice rota system of out-of-hours care with a deputising service, showed a slightly increased level of satisfaction with the practice-based service (70 per cent) compared with deputising service (61 per cent). Deputising doctors were more likely to prescribe, but there was no difference in rates of hospital admission.[27]

**Out-of-hours general practice and palliative care**

Little is published regarding out-of-hours palliative care in general

---

Box 2.1 **Benefits of belonging to an out-of-hours cooperative (NAGPC)**

---

- Offers an efficient use of GPs' time on call out of hours.

- The members are principals on a Health Authority (PCT) list and, as they are directly responsible for their own actions, the general standard of care provided by a GP cooperative should be as good as that of other general medical services in the area.

- The doctors are local GPs; they will be committed to maintaining high standards on behalf of their GP colleagues.

- A GP cooperative is democratically run; its service is responsive to the needs of the local population and local GPs.

- Patients can have confidence in a service run and staffed by local GPs.

- The costs of running a GP cooperative should be lower than a commercial deputising service because it cannot and does not make a profit.

- Local GPs provide the service – their knowledge of local health services ensures that these facilities are used effectively.

- Local GPs share a common commitment to constraining inappropriate demands for out-of-hours care.

- A GP cooperative can normally allow each GP member to choose how much to use the service and how much they might offer to do for the service, although some may choose to operate a compulsory shift system.

- In many areas cooperatives have become a focus for wider social, professional and educational contact within the GP community and have undoubtedly improved morale among GPs in their localities.

- As cooperatives are groups of local GPs, a bid can be made for some operating costs to the Out of Hours Development Fund (OOHDF).

*Source*: National Association of GP Co-operatives.[22]

practice before 1995. The advent of cooperatives did lead to concerns on the part of opinion leaders and organisations interested in palliative care.[28,29] With the lack of previous studies it is difficult to ascertain whether care for palliative care patients was of a poorer quality in cooperatives than it had been before, although it might be argued that GPs working in rota arrangements within and between practices were more likely to know of a palliative care patient, either directly or through informal briefing by colleagues. How this translated into quality of care, however, is largely speculative.

### Issues of concern: communication

The first published study of out-of-hours palliative care described the results of an audit undertaken in an English cooperative, which surveyed the contacts with palliative care patients over a one-month period in 1996.[30] Of 2202 contacts, 53 were for 40 patients identifiably in the terminal phase of their illness, i.e. 2 per cent of all patient contacts. There was no evidence that the registered GP had handed over information for any of these patients. In most cases the attending doctor for those patients who had more than one contact with the cooperative had no information regarding the patient's previous contact. Also, the GP with whom the patient was registered mainly received notification of the visit by post, rather than by fax or electronic means. The conclusion of the authors was that the cooperative

> seems not to function well with terminally ill patients, who constituted a small but important part of its workload. If primary care is to remain central to palliative and terminal care every effort must be made to minimise the adverse impact of the recent changes in out of hours care.[30]

In a similar audit of palliative care out of hours in a Scottish cooperative, it was found that for palliative care patients identified by district nurses over a period of one month as being terminally ill (defined as likely to be within one month of death), 5/24 (21 per cent) had a notification sent to the cooperative regarding the patient by their GP. Although this represented a small number of patients within a cooperative serving a population of 300,000, examining cooperative records suggested that for 75 per cent of these patients a call to the cooperative had been made.[31] Data therefore from these two audits suggest that, although the number of calls for palliative care patients represented only a small proportion of the total calls to these cooperatives, palliative care patients are in fact probably highly likely to call out of hours. These data have been supported by the results of other studies.[32,33]

### Exploring issues of communication

Communication regarding palliative care patients between GPs and out-of-hours providers is rightly regarded as an important aspect of good practice,[34-6] particularly because such patients are likely to need to seek help out of hours, have complex needs and they and their carers are likely to be in a state of extreme stress. Evidence suggests that patients and carers feel reassured by knowing that out-of-hours professional carers have received information from their usual healthcare professionals (see Chapter 5). However, whether such necessarily limited information in a potentially rapidly changing clinical situation leads GPs to deliver superior care in the out-of-hours period in practice is an area in need of further research.

Gilroy, a cooperative general manager, undertook a study exploring the effects of communication within his cooperative.[32] Over a one-month period a total of 3261 calls were received, of which 24 (0.7 per cent) were for 15 palliative care patients. Over half of the contacts had been regarding pain control, one had been to confirm death and the others were recorded as being for a variety of symptom issues. Sixteen calls had resulted in home visits, seven in telephone advice and one patient attended the Primary Care Centre of the cooperative. For each of the 24 calls a questionnaire was sent to the attending GP and 20 of these were returned. For none of these patients was written information from the GP available within the cooperative, despite a system for communication being available; however, the attending GP recorded that they were able to access information in addition to that given by the patient or carer on 13 occasions. Apart from information gained from previous contact with the cooperative on one occasion and the patient's GP on another, the commonest source of information was from community nursing notes left within the patient's home or from direct contact with a community specialist nurse.

GPs were asked to indicate whether in their opinion further information could have altered the final outcome or improved their standard of response in the particular clinical situation. For three calls GPs indicated that further information could have improved the care given, 15 felt that it would not have made a difference and for two cases the GP was unsure. For none of these patients did the encounter result in hospital admission.

Whilst in approximately half of the clinical encounters, more information on the patient's medical history or the extent of the patient's or carer's knowledge of their condition was considered to have been potentially useful, knowledge of the patient's social circumstances, availability of lay carer or professional support were considered to have been less important. In this study GPs did not feel that for most situations they had difficulty in controlling the patient's symptoms as a result of a lack of information and no GP indicated that they had more than 'some difficulty' in controlling symptoms. Gilroy concluded that his study illustrated Cook's assertion that 'in practice, gaps in continuity of care, such as lack of information, rarely lead to overt failure'.[37] Rather than claiming that communication was unimportant, Gilroy argued that it illustrated how GPs in the real world were able to overcome lack of information in a variety of ways.

In a parallel interview study by Gilroy,[32] with a subset of five GPs who had completed the questionnaire, GPs indicated what potentially important information regarding palliative care patients was needed in advance. This would include:

- details of medical history
- details of diagnosis and current management
- details of patient and family knowledge, and understanding regarding their disease.

In addition, some interviewees indicated that lack of information could be sensitively handled by careful interviewing of the patient and their carer, and giving them time and attention, illustrating how their skill as GPs could be effectively used in difficult and sensitive situations. Conversely, some suggested that having information regarding patients would enable them to avoid the situation of the patient or carer having to go through the heartache of recounting the story to a stranger, and would lessen their need to rely on the relative's account of the patient's condition, which they felt was not always reliable.

### Improving out-of-hours palliative care

When asked about how out-of-hours palliative care could be improved, the GPs interviewed did not make negative comments about their colleagues' lack of communication with the cooperative regarding palliative care patients, but they were critical of colleagues' failure to ensure adequate care was given in hours, which led to an out-of-hours crisis. Whilst all GPs agreed that information regarding palliative care patients was desirable, some of the GPs pointed out that faxed information could become rapidly out of date. Information kept within the patient's home would be possibly more reliable and up to date. All agreed that moves toward an electronic health record, available out of hours, was highly desirable, but they were less than hopeful that this could become a reality.

Gilroy's study, although based on a small number of participants, gives useful insights into how GPs working out of hours may use their skill and experience to overcome issues regarding lack of information. The study also uses the theoretical work of Cook to show how professionals can bridge gaps in knowledge by relying on their technical and professional skills. He also highlights the important issue of the rapidity with which information can become unreliable because the clinical situation has progressed.

The importance of this study is that it illustrates how quality of out-of-hours care cannot be simply equated with the presence or absence of information sent from the usual carer regarding the patient. It is possible for GPs to practise effectively despite a lack of information, and quality of care may be related more to the GP's clinical and communication skills, and a sensitive, caring approach.

Wendy-Jane Walton's personal view (Chapter 3) illustrates how an experienced, skilled and caring GP can provide high-quality out-of-hours care for dying patients in the community. Also, insights gained from the Scottish study into patient experience out of hours (Chapter 5) illustrate how effective and sensitive communication by the GP to patients and carers is an important element in providing care, for which patients and their carers express high levels of satisfaction.

## Overview of palliative care activity with cooperatives

Communicating information regarding a patient with complex needs who is also likely to call is normally considered best practice. It is, however, also vital that the information is available when a call is received regarding the patient. Many cooperatives use IT systems and some use this to 'flag up' the fact that information is available regarding a patient when a call is received. The call handler receiving the call is alerted to the fact that this call is regarding a palliative care patient and is able to locate the information and make it available to the GP dealing with the call.

Some cooperatives seemingly independently designed fax forms to facilitate transfer of relevant information regarding palliative care patients. Others developed protocols for palliative care,[38] provided special education in palliative care for their members and audited their activity. Such examples of good practice were emerging from individual cooperatives (Box 2.2); however, little was known of the general situation. In an attempt to gain this wider picture, a survey of 133 medical directors of cooperatives throughout the UK was undertaken in 1999 at the University of Warwick.[39] The majority (81 per cent) reported that a system existed within the cooperative to enable GP practices to send information to the cooperative regarding patients for whom the GP judged there was a need. Relatively few cooperatives used dedicated fax forms (20 per cent) designed to capture important patient information or used computer systems (29 per cent) to alert cooperative staff to the fact that information regarding a patient was available if a call was received.

GP facilitators in palliative care, whose aim is to enable the delivery of high-quality palliative care in the primary care setting, were reported to be available for 39/133 (30 per cent) but interestingly had been used by only 14 co-operatives. Not surprisingly where the services of the facilitators were employed, cooperatives were more likely to demonstrate activity around audit, educational events and specific palliative care protocols and equipment (see Table 2.1).

Table 2.1 **Palliative care organisation in co-operatives – according to medical director**

|  | With facilitator input | Without facilitator input |  |
|---|---|---|---|
| Audit of Palliative Care | 3/14 (21%) | 5/119 (4%) | $p = 0.015^*$ |
| Equipment or Protocols | 8/14 (57%) | 31/119 (26%) | $\chi^2 = 5.84, p = 0.015$ |
| Education in Palliative Care | 3/14 (21%) | 7/119 (6%) | $p = 0.030^*$ |

*Fisher exact test as number <5

---

Box 2.2 **Examples of good practice from individual cooperatives**

---

**'Bearder' bags**

These were developed in the Calderdale and Kirklees Health Authority for use by cooperative and deputising services. They are specially assembled bags that contain:

- syringe driver
- crisis packs with symptom control guidelines and contact details
- palliative care drugs, syringes and needles.

These bags are available in the cooperative cars and deputising service bases. The bags are supported by a local charity in memory of Mr John Bearder.

**Grampian Doctors on Call**

*Established 1996*

- GP Palliative Care Facilitator provided a list of palliative care drugs to be carried in 'doctor's' bags.

*1997–8*

- Audit performed to assess whether GPs communicated with the co-op regarding terminally ill patients.
- Results of initial audit led to introduction of fax form. Adopted unanimously by co-op membership.
- Re-audit demonstrated an improvement in levels of communication.

*1999*

- GP Palliative Care Facilitator conducted an audit on symptom control measures taken by visiting doctors.
- An educational event was arranged and very well attended by the membership. Afternoon session devoted to palliative care issues.

---

This lack of activity is interesting and perhaps reflects the fact that palliative care represents only a small proportion of cooperative activity and therefore was not seen as a high priority within the cooperative, rather than cooperatives seeing palliative care as being unimportant. Also it is possible that activity within cooperatives generally increased following this survey, although more recent studies have indicated little change in practice regarding communication.[33]

### GP and district nurse (DN) satisfaction with out-of-hours general practice for palliative care

A questionnaire study in 2000 from King's College London,[40] of 715 GPs and 317 DNs in seven health districts in a variety of settings, ranging from inner-city to urban and rural locations, surveyed out-of-hours GP service provision for palliative care patients and satisfaction with such services. Almost three-quarters of GPs responding indicated that they were members of cooperatives, one-fifth provided practice based on call, whilst only one in 20 GPs used deputising services. Only 23 per cent indicated that they handed over all of their out-of-hours care for palliative care patients with the majority indicating that they provided personal care at least some of the time to terminally ill patients. Most GPs were satisfied with their out-of-hours arrangements, whilst few were highly satisfied. Notably, inner-city GPs were less satisfied than urban or rural GPs. DNs were less satisfied than GPs with out-of-hours GP arrangements, citing dissatisfaction with the quality of some advice, a reluctance to visit, and difficulties in obtaining medication. GPs' dissatisfaction was particularly with having to care for patients whom they did not know.

### Issues of concern: GPs and the availability of specialist services out of hours

Both of these surveys reviewed GP experiences and attitudes to the availability of specialist services out of hours. The King's study found that 60 per cent of GPs wanted access to specialist palliative care advice out of hours. The Warwick study found that, whilst 94 per cent of respondents reported the availability of specialist palliative care services 'in hours', 37 per cent believed they had access to specialist advice, and 31 per cent access to specialist beds out of hours. Satisfaction with specialist advice was rated as high or moderate by 88 per cent of those with access to it. However, several comments suggested that since the need for it was so infrequent it was difficult to rate its quality. Some negative comments suggested that at times advice was only available from a junior staff member, which was not considered appropriate, or that there was difficulty in contacting the appropriate person.

The Warwick cooperative study was accompanied by a parallel review of hospice and specialist palliative care units which reported that 89 per cent of hospices offered an advice service to GPs.[39] For the cooperatives that could be matched with a responding specialist palliative care unit, in only half was there concordance, with cooperative and palliative care unit medical directors agreeing that specialist palliative care advice out of hours was available. In the other half, whilst a service was provided by the hospice, the cooperative medical director indicated that they lacked awareness of it, despite most hospices claiming to have informed GPs of the service.

The majority (71 per cent) of GP cooperative medical directors surveyed wanted access to specialist palliative care beds out of hours. However, comments suggested that admission to palliative care beds out of hours was rarely needed. In addition some indicated that since beds are normally full during working hours it seemed pointless trying to admit a patient out of hours. Hence, patients needing in-patient care were normally admitted into general hospital beds.

**Recent changes: new GP contract**

In June 2003 GPs voted for a new contract that had been negotiated on their behalf by the General Practice Committee of the British Medical Association. One major change was that GPs would no longer be required to provide 24-hour care for their registered patients, but could 'opt out' of providing such a service. The provision of out-of-hours medical services when the new contract was introduced became the responsibility of the Primary Care Trust (PCT). The new contract came into force in April 2004, although in some PCTs the new out-of-hours arrangements were not put into place until December 2004.

Whilst GP out-of-hours arrangements since 1995 had been moving largely towards cooperatives and away from practice-based and deputising services, the new arrangements are likely to be highly variable with no 'typical' service configuration. Some PCTs have no GP home visits, with triage being conducted over the telephone backed up by specifically trained paramedical staff or 'Emergency Care Practitioners' (ECP). In these PCTs, patients needing to have medical assessment either attend an out-of-hours centre, A&E, or are admitted directly to hospital, depending on clinical need. Other PCTs have maintained GP visiting services, albeit normally at reduced availability. Two factors are likely to have reduced the availability of GPs out of hours. The first is that a relatively low proportion of GPs are prepared to work out of hours since the inception of the new contract,[41] and the second is that there is a potential lack of funding available to PCTs; GPs in opting out of out-of-hours care had their NHS incomes reduced by approximately £6000, which probably represents only a fraction of the cost of providing the GP services to the pre-new contract level.[42]

How primary palliative care services will be maintained is not clear. Some examples of good practices are emerging (see Box 2.3); however, it is clear that some PCTs are finding it difficult to provide robust services within the cost constraints that exist. A concern must be that PCTs will not be able to afford services that will be appropriate for palliative care patients and the quality of care will reduce, with patients needing to wait for long periods for a doctor to visit,

---

**Box 2.3 South Warwickshire PCT – out-of-hours palliative care**

No GPs are on duty out of hours to provide home visits in South Warwickshire, an area covering a 236,000 population in three urban centres (Warwick – Leamington Spa, Stratford-upon-Avon and Kenilworth) and a large rural area stretching into the Cotswold Hills in the south. Visits are performed by ECPs – either from a nursing or a paramedic background. Patients needing to see a doctor are seen at the out-of-hours centre, based at Warwick Hospital, or admitted to hospital.

In order to provide an enhanced service for palliative care patients, a rota of eight GPs has been established to give advice and, if necessary, a home visit to these patients. Calls are triaged through the out-of-hours service and passed to the palliative care GP if appropriate.

Early indications are that the service is well accepted by patients, carers and health professionals. On average, one call is received in the course of one week of nights and two to four calls at the weekend. It is also felt to be effective in preventing admission to hospital.

An arrangement has been made with local pharmacists to provide a list of essential drugs out of hours. Specialist advice is available from on-call clinical nurse specialists and consultants in palliative medicine. Admission to the hospice is sometimes available out of hours following discussion between the palliative care GP and the consultant on call.

being inappropriately forced to attend out-of-hours centres or being admitted to hospital. However, the new arrangements could provide an opportunity to develop improved services, with out-of-hours primary care staff receiving special training in palliative care accompanied by an enhanced specialist advice service, as recommended by the National Institute for Health and Clinical Excellence (NICE) Guidance for Supportive and Palliative Care.[43] What is clear is that out-of-hours palliative care in the community demands a well coordinated, skilled, responsive and flexible service for a relatively small number of patients. If it is not made a priority for funding based on a compassionate approach, rather than an overemphasis on efficiency, aspirations for high-quality care will not be realised.

## Conclusions

The British system of providing universal primary care services 24 hours a day, every day of the year, has undergone extensive change in the past 10 years, not least in how out-of-hours care is provided. After 1995, out-of-hours cooperatives rapidly became the commonest system for delivering GP services; however, the direction has radically altered following the adoption of the new GP contract in April 2004 when GPs could opt out of providing 24-hour care for their patients.

Providing continuity of care into the out-of-hours period is a complex issue, and not merely one of ensuring that forward planning for patients' care occurs or that information is passed onto out-of-hours providers. Out-of-hours providers need to be effectively resourced, organised and trained to provide an adequate standard of palliative care. General practitioners have traditionally provided out-of-hours primary care and are skilled at managing complex problems in less than ideal circumstances. As the population ages and increasing numbers of patients with chronic cancer and non-cancer illnesses with complicated co-morbidities live in the community, such skills will be increasingly needed to ensure patients are managed appropriately and safely.

Despite some evidence for deficiencies in delivery of palliative care by GPs in the out-of-hours period, there is no clear evidence that alternative systems would be superior. It is likely that general practitioners will continue to be a vital source of skill for out-of-hours primary palliative care if appropriate and sustainable levels of care are to be maintained.

### *Acknowledgement*

We would like to thank Dr Rodger Charlton who gave valuable advice for a draft of this chapter.

## Summary

- Out-of-hours general practice has undergone radical change in the last 10 years.

- Communication of information from GP to the out-of-hours provider is an important aspect of good practice. Information, however, may rapidly become out of date.

- Good communication and clinical skills are vital for GPs providing out-of-hours care.

- Gaps in information may be overcome by a GP's experience and skill in dealing with uncertainty.

- The new GP contract may have detrimental effects on out-of-hours palliative care; conversely it may provide opportunities for enhancing care.

## REFERENCES

1. Olesen F, Dickinson J and Hjortdahl P. General practice – Time for a new definition. *British Medical Journal* 2000; **320 (7231)**: 354–7.

2. Freeman G K, Olesen F and Hjortdahl P. Continuity of care: An essential element of modern general practice? *Family Practice* 2003; **20 (6)**: 623–7.

3. Schers H, Webster S, van den Hoogen H, Avery A, Grohl R and van den Bosch W. Continuity of care in general practice: A survey of patients' views. *British Journal of General Practice* 2002; **52**: 459–62.

4. Heath I. *The Mystery of General Practice*. London: Nuffield Provincial Hospitals Trust, 1995.

5. Kearley K, Freeman G and Heath A. An exploration of the value of the personal doctor–patient relationship in general practice. *British Journal of General Practice* 2001; **51**: 712–18.

6. Field D. Special not different: General practitioners' accounts of their care of dying people. *Social Science and Medicine* 1998; **46 (9)**: 1111–20.

7. Jessopp L, Beck I, Hollins L, Shipman C, Reynolds M and Dale J. Changing the pattern out of hours: A survey of general practice cooperatives. *British Medical Journal* 1997; **314 (7075)**: 199.

8. Fakhoury W, McCarthy M and Addington-Hall J. The effects of the clinical characteristics of dying cancer patients on informal caregivers' satisfaction with palliative care. *Palliative Medicine* 1997; **11**: 107–15.

9. Barclay S, Todd C J, Grande G and Lipscombe J. How common is medical training in palliative care? A postal survey of general practitioners. *British Journal of General Practice* 1997; **47**: 800–5.

10. Grande G, Barclay S and Todd C J. Difficulty of symptom control and general practitioners' knowledge of patients' symptoms. *Palliative Medicine* 1997; **11**: 399–406.

11. *The GP Palliative Care Facilitator Project*. London: Royal College of General Practitioners, 1995.

12. Department of Health. *Investing in General Practice: The new general medical services contract*. London: Department of Health, 2003.

13. Salisbury C. Visiting through the night. *British Medical Journal* 1993; **306**: 762–4.

14. Hallam L. Primary medical care outside normal working hours: Review of published work. *British Medical Journal* 1994; **308 (6923)**: 249–53.

15. Salisbury C and Boerma W. Balancing demand and supply in out-of-hours care. In: Salisbury C, Dale J and Hallam L, eds. *24 Hour Primary Care*. Oxford: Radcliffe Medical, 1999, pp. 17–31.

16. Electoral Reform Ballot Services. *Your Choices for the Future: A survey of GP opinion, UK report*. London: Electoral Reform Ballot Services, 1992.

17. Hurwitz B. The new out of hours agreement for general practitioners. *British Medical Journal* 1995; **311 (7009)**: 824–5.

18. National Association of GP Co-operatives. *Co-ops and the NAGPC* [web page]. 1995; available at: www.nagpc.org.uk/nonmembers/nmcoopsnagpc.htm [accessed March 2007].

19. Hallam L and Reynolds M. GP out of hours co-operatives. In: Salisbury C, Dale J and Hallam L, eds. *24 Hour Primary Care*. Oxford: Radcliffe Medical, 1999, pp. 63–91.

20. Salisbury C. Evaluation of a general practice out of hours co-operative: A questionnaire survey of general practitioners. *British Medical Journal* 1997; **314**: 1598.

21. Hughes P, Neal R D and Maskrey N. General practitioners prefer to work in cooperatives for out of hours work. *British Medical Journal* 1997; **314 (7098)**: 1904.

22. National Association of GP Co-operatives. *Characteristics of a GP co-operative* [web page]. Available at www.nagpc.org.uk/nonmembers/nmcoopcharcteristics.htm [accessed March 2007].

23. Salisbury C. Postal survey of patients' satisfaction with a general practice out of hours co-operative. *British Medical Journal* 1997; **314**: 1594–8.

24. Shipman C, Payne F, Hooper R and Dale J. Patients' satisfaction with out of hours services; How do GP co-operatives compare with deputising and practice based arrangements? *Journal of Public Health Medicine* 2000; **22**: 149–54.

25. Leibowitz R, Day S and Dunt D. A systematic review of the effect of different models of after-hours primary medical services on clinical outcome, medical workload and patient and GP satisfaction. *Family Practice* 2003; **20**: 311–17.

26. McKinley R K, Cragg D K, Hastings A M, *et al.* Comparison of out of hours care provided by patients' own general practitioners and commercial deputising services: A randomised controlled trial. II: The outcome of care. *British Medical Journal* 1997; **314 (7075)**: 190.

27. Cragg D K, McKinley R K, Roland M O, *et al.* Comparison of out of hours care provided by patients' own general practitioners and commercial deputising services: A randomised controlled trial. I: The process of care. *British Medical Journal* 1997; **314 (7075)**: 187.

28. Scottish Cancer Coordinating and Advisory Committee. *Commissioning Cancer Services in Scotland, Primary and Palliative Care Services – Report to the Chief Medical Officer*. Scottish Office Department of Health, 1997.

29. Barclay S. palliative care in the community: The role of the primary care team. *Palliative Care Today* 1998; **6**: 46–7.

30. Barclay S, Rogers M and Todd C. Communication between GPs and cooperatives is poor for terminally ill patients. *British Medical Journal* 1997; **315**: 1235 b–6.

31. Munday D, Carroll D and Douglas A. GP out of hours co-operatives and the delivery of palliative care. *British Journal of General Practice* 1999; **49**: 489.

32. Gilroy J. What are the difficulties caused by a lack of patient information when co-operative duty doctors receive a request for palliative care during the out of hours period? [MSc dissertation]. Coventry: University of Warwick, 2001.

33. Burt J, Barclay S, Marshall N, Shipman C, Stimson A and Young J. Continuity within primary care: An audit of general practice out of hours co-operatives. *Journal of Public Health* 2004; **26**: 275–6.

34. Higginson I. Who needs palliative care? *Journal of the Royal Society of Medicine* 1998; **91**: 563–4.

35. Thomas K. *Out of Hours Palliative Care in the Community*. London: Macmillan Cancer Relief, 2001.

36. *Raising Standards for Patients: New partnerships in out of hours care*. London: Department of Health, 2000.

37. Cook R I, Render M and Woods D. Gaps in the continuity of care and progress on patient safety. *British Medical Journal* 2000; **320**: 791–4.

38. King N, Thomas K and Bell D. An out of hours protocol for community palliative care: Practitioners' perspectives. *International Journal of Palliative Nursing* 2003; **9**: 277–82.

39. Munday D, Dale J and Barnett M. Out of hours palliative care in the UK: Perspectives from general practice and specialist services. *Journal of the Royal Society of Medicine* 2002; **95**: 28–30.

40. Shipman C, Addington-Hall J, Barclay S, *et al*. Providing palliative care in primary care: How satisfied are GPs and district nurses with current out of hours arrangements? *British Journal of General Practice* 2000; **50 (455)**: 477–8.

41. Koralage N. GPs reluctant to cover out of hours work, survey shows. *British Medical Journal* 2004; **328 (7434)**: 247 a.

42. Mayor S. Report warns that cost of care by GPs out of hours could be higher than expected. *British Medical Journal* 2004; **329**: 368.

43. *Guidance on Cancer Services: Improving supportive and palliative care for adults*. London: National Institute for Clinical Excellence, 2004.

CHAPTER | 3

# A GP's personal view

'On dying'

*Wendy-Jane Walton*

---

I am writing this about two hours after receiving the news that my close friend and colleague, Dr Steve Hugh, Medical Manager of Shropdoc, has died suddenly in Spain. I am numb with shock and disbelief; he was several years shy of 50, married with two children, energetic, active and utterly committed to his work of spearheading the GP out-of-hours service in Shropshire.

I had been thinking of Steve quite a bit this weekend, anyway, after a particularly satisfying clinical session in the Shropdoc car on Saturday morning. Since the Primary Care Trusts (PCTs) took over responsibility for out-of-hours cover in October 2004, Shropdoc has provided an effective and reliable service for the patients of Shropshire, and across its borders into Wales and surrounding counties. It has continued to run on a very similar model to that which was in operation prior to the new contract, albeit with slimmed down numbers of doctors on clinical shifts, and an expansion of the triage operation to include specially trained nurses.

Other PCTs, in an effort to keep costs to a minimum, have adopted other solutions, including using the ambulance service, walk-in centres and nurse-led services, but my experiences on Saturday morning left me pondering that there are many situations in which there is no substitute for the clinical experience and training of a GP.

The first two calls were to elderly ladies in nursing homes, both of whom had 'collapsed'. The first was a tiny, bird-like woman with a barely detectable pulse and a clinical picture of widespread sepsis against a background of progressive deterioration and frailty. She was being comfortably nursed, was not in pain or agitated and was able to take sips of fluid but not her usual medication. Following discussion with the nursing staff and family it was agreed that she should be kept comfortable and allowed to slip away peacefully. The second was an almost identical situation in another nursing home, where the woman's daughters had already prepared to set up vigil by her bedside. Her medication list ran to four pages and included expensive antidepressants and antihypertensives as well as morphine tablets and suspension. As she was unable to swallow any tablets it was decided that these could be omitted and her pain relief covered with morphine suspension. In both cases all parties were in accord that hospital admission would be inappropriate, that death was the likely outcome, and that resuscitation should not be attempted. Of the six other cases I visited that morning, only one, which had also been logged as a 'collapse' of an elderly lady living alone, required admission, for management of a urinary tract infection with newly presenting diabetes. I was able to make the diagnosis and admit direct to a medical bed. The others were easily managed at home; one was a catheter change in a young man with severe end-stage motor neurone disease who would otherwise have had to wait until the district nurses picked up their messages in the afternoon. In some cases I was able to prescribe or administer medication, and in all to allay anxiety. The five hours flew by, and I realised that I had accomplished more real medicine than I sometimes see in a whole week in surgery. Had a GP not been available to these people, the alternatives for almost all of them would have been transportation to hospital and a long wait for assessment in A&E, since nurses and paramedics do not have the clinical training to diagnose and treat. The costs saved by keeping people in the community are substantial, not to mention the obvious benefits to the patient of being able to remain in his or her home environment.

As a GP registrar almost 20 years ago I gained my out-of-hours experience by participating in the training practice rota, learning the hard way, on the hoof, on my own, without the benefit of a driver or a mobile phone. Looking back now it seems almost foolhardy, and was without a doubt stressful, particularly since the concept of triage was not established and almost everything got a visit, but it has stood me in good stead, and, as my trainer memorably said, we should all work out of hours since many problems 'come home to roost in the middle of the night'.

I am concerned that current GP registrars get far less training and experience in out-of-hours work than used to be the case, and wonder how this will impact upon the medical staffing of services in the future, since it is no longer a requirement of the GP contract. Good rates of pay may attract younger doctors to out of hours, but will PCTs be able to maintain the budgets for these services? Can they afford not to?

One of the areas of major concern is the care of the dying, with a move towards enabling all dying patients, whatever their diagnosis, to be cared for, and if possible to die, in their place of choice. For many people this will mean additional resources being required to enable them to remain at home, and GPs will be called upon increasingly to implement their skills and knowledge of patients and their families in providing the palliative care that these patients need, in cooperation, of course, with community nursing teams and Specialist Palliative Care Services, as well as the out-of-hours service. Since out of hours represents over two-thirds of the working week, communication between services about patient care plans is critical. The Gold Standards Framework[1] in palliative care is one tool that is being widely used across the country to ensure that dying patients in the community are given the best possible care, and inappropriate crisis admissions avoided.

What I do know is that when I am old (if I am granted such longevity) and if my dying is predictable, I should like to be confident that I can be cared for in a place where I feel safe and secure, with people around me whom I know and trust. I would like my symptoms to be well controlled, as I know is perfectly possible with available medication, but I do not want to be given large numbers of unnecessary drugs. I do not want to be removed to a hospital for want of available care at home, and I do not want to be artificially kept alive or resuscitated when death is inevitable. I certainly do not want to live out my final days under the shadow of a possibility that a well-intentioned healthcare professional may undertake to hasten or assist my dying. I believe we go down that road at our peril.

Steve Hugh was passionately committed to the model of GP cooperatives as the nucleus of a high-quality, multidisciplinary out-of-hours service, and as we mourn our colleague I know that we should consider carefully our role in caring for those who are expected to die. The introduction of Advance Decisions, clear instructions regarding resuscitation status and care plans for the dying, should help in determining and communicating patients' needs. We should be prepared to talk about these sensitive issues with our patients, communicate their wishes, and ensure that they do not fall foul of a second-rate service when the surgery is closed.

### Acknowledgement

This chapter is reprinted from the *Midlands Faculty News* of the Royal College of General Practitioners (December 2005) with the kind permission of the editor.

**REFERENCE**

1. www.goldstandardsframework.nhs.uk [accessed March 2007].

CHAPTER | 4

# District nurses and continuity of palliative care

*Cathy Shipman, Allison Worth and Jenni Burt*

## Introduction

In this chapter we look at the role of the district nursing service in providing continuity of palliative care to patients and families. District and community nurses (DNs) are pivotal to palliative care in the community and we shall describe the central role that DN teams play in supporting palliative care patients and carers to remain at home for as long as is possible and desired. We shall also discuss some key issues that impact on the delivery of community nursing care both within and out of hours, and look at examples of good practice.

The main issues will be illustrated using examples from two studies, first a study of out-of-hours palliative care in Scotland, conducted in 2001 to 2003,[1] and second a study of Primary Care Trusts (PCTs) commissioning and providing palliative care across London in 2004.[2] Both provide different perspectives on the service. The Scottish study was of specialist palliative care nurses, district nurses and Marie Curie and other nurses working in a range of roles with palliative care patients out of hours. This study also included a survey of all out-of-hours nursing services (19) in Scotland including the perspectives of other professionals, such as GPs, on community nursing, as well as those of patient and carer. The London study sought the views of district nurses, GPs and other healthcare professionals about palliative care provision in five London Primary Care Trusts (PCTs).[2]

**District and community nursing teams providing palliative care**

DNs have long been identified as the key healthcare professionals providing hands-on nursing care to patients at home.[3] The majority of palliative care patients at home receive care at some point from a DN team, and, whilst the extent of palliative care provision to patients can vary, at times such care comprises a substantial part of DN work.[4] A recent study across five London PCTs found that 91.8 per cent (167/182) of responding DNs said that they were currently providing palliative care, in comparison with 65.9 per cent (232/352) of GPs.[2] DNs reported caring, on average, for five palliative care patients, whilst GPs reported caring for two. Visiting patients increasingly frequently towards the end of life, members of DN teams are often best placed to assess changes in symptom control needs. They frequently take on a coordinating role, referring to Marie Cure nurses and social services, seeking the support of specialist palliative care nurses and reporting on patient progress to GPs. This role was set out in the government's nursing strategy for the NHS – *Making a Difference*[5] – as central to enabling patients to remain at home, with nurses acting as 'patient assessors, care-co-ordinators and team leaders'. This role was further highlighted by the Community Practitioners and Health Visitors Association (CPVA) briefing – *District Nursing at the Crossroads*[6] – and strengthened by the Department of Health-funded Education and Support Programme in Palliative Care across England.[7] DNs themselves recognise the centrality of their role in palliative care.[2]

**Continuity of care**

Theoretical aspects of continuity of care have been described within the introductory chapter. In an extensive review of literature Haggerty *et al.* suggest that, within primary care, longitudinal, relational or personal continuity has been most prominent, 'viewed as the relationship between a single practitioner and a patient that extends beyond specific episodes of disease'. Within nursing literature, however, the focus has been on the coordination of care over time and information transfer, with a particular emphasis on discharge planning following acute care.[8]

While district nurses are not likely to have contact with patients and carers over a lifetime, when providing palliative care their involvement can be more extensive than that of other health and social care providers. Increased home visiting towards the end of life can foster the development of personal continuity, continuity over time and, if sufficient resources and support are accessible, in many cases continuity of place of care. In terms of Haggerty's criteria, as coordinators of care, district nurses are centrally involved in supporting informational, management and relational continuity whether they remain the key contact for the patient or not. In providing hands-on nursing care, they are frequently assessing symptom control needs and liaising with GPs or specialist palliative care, providing informational continuity. As a coordinator of service input they are well placed to support management continuity, and often, as the most frequent visitor to the home, provide relational continuity, a point also developed within the chapter on patient experiences. To achieve continuity of care on this scale, however, district nursing teams need sufficient time and resources to be able to spend enough time in the patient's home to provide nursing and supportive care. They also need to be able to access services and support from other health and social care professionals when needed.

The patient need for continuity of care, however, does not stop at the end of the working day. Within this chapter we shall therefore also consider continuity in terms of access to 24-hour care. This is particularly important because access to district nursing outside the normal working week is frequently limited and in some instances non-existent. Informational, management and relational (where possible) continuity are important for the effective seamless delivery of 24-hour care.

## Threats to continuity of palliative care

### Access to health and social services

Good availability and easy access to key health and social care services is essential to enable patients to be supported at home. Effective coordination of these services makes a major contribution to continuity of care. However, availability and access to other services and professionals involved in palliative care provision – including GP home visits, specialist palliative care nurses, Marie Curie nurses and respite care – is reported by DNs to be variable. A national survey of DNs' perceptions of access to support services found that, although most considered access to GP home visits and specialist palliative care assessment was at least usually available, only just over half thought that this was always available.[9] For about 40 per cent of DNs, Marie or other night-sitting service were at best only sometimes available. Whilst not all palliative care patients will need support from specialist services, most will need some GP home visits, and thus reliable access to these is essential. Accessibility of services is particularly important to carers,[10] with increased frequency of visits from DNs, contact with other services, the provision of help at night and perceived sufficient knowledge of the circumstances and care needs of the patients all being associated with higher carer satisfaction.[11,12]

In the Scottish study[1] support for carers, from nursing, social care or non-statutory services, was seen as vital to the successful provision of out-of-hours palliative care. Such support was generally supplied by unqualified staff, some with palliative care training, and included sitting with patients overnight to allow exhausted carers some sleep/respite and providing carers with emotional support and a link to trained nurses, if needed. Availability of such care was perceived as patchy, declining and described by professionals as inequitable and inadequate to meet patient needs and carer expectations. It was seen as a major factor in breaking down palliative care at home out of hours, and as probably contributing to inappropriate admissions to hospital:

> The main problem is that there are not sufficient services for people to be cared for at home … maybe a breakdown in carers because they don't get enough respite.
>
> (Community hospital nurse, rural area)

Rural areas appeared to have a particular problem, in that both Marie Curie and social workers required a considerable period of notice in order to make a commitment to provide night care, yet need for the service was unpredictable and help was rarely available in an emergency. As one carer said:

> when I asked the district nurse if I could have a night nurse when

my husband was at that last week of his life, and they said 'oh well no it'll take four days to organise'.

In addition, carers were rarely able to access all the help they needed, so that they might request seven nights' care but receive only three. For people without informal carers, 24-hour care at home was perceived as virtually impossible to organise at the end of life. This was apparent to patients and carers.

Less than half the cooperatives in Scotland reported 24-hour access to telephone advice from a specialist palliative care doctor or nurse. Some professionals suggested that specialist care should be available out of hours, but others that demand was insufficient to warrant this and a more formalised system of advice provision was preferable. Some patients and carers expressed a preference for specialist palliative care advice out of hours, one carer saying:

my problem is there is nobody I can call for palliative care out of hours ... and that's something I really would like looked at ... the doctors have all been good ... the nurses have all been good, but I just have an anxiety that they are generalists and they are not specialists in palliative care.

Provision of specialist advice was sometimes dependent on individual nurses acting outside their normal working times:

I have had on occasion, where I have real concerns, contacted whoever is on for the out-of-hours service in that evening and said 'I know this gentleman well. If this happens then I feel that he would wish admission just perhaps to a specific ward, or he would wish to remain at home', so that I have addressed that directly with whoever is on that evening.

(Macmillan nurse)

## Early and appropriate referral

Early referral to DN teams is important to enable the development of a therapeutic relationship with the patient and carer,[13,14] and the experience of continuity of care. Early referrals from GPs are a key preference for district nursing services as identified in the Scottish study[1] where DNs expressed a need for earlier information from

GPs on people who are likely to need their support in the later stages of illness. They described the difficulties associated with only meeting the patient and family for the first time a few days before death.

However, the Audit Commission survey found that one in ten of all referrals to district nursing services was felt to be inappropriate.[15] Many DNs did not feel able to control referrals and were only able to manage their caseloads by changing the frequency and duration of their visits. This has clear implications for the provision of palliative care, which requires more frequent and longer visits to deal with more urgent, serious and often complex problems.

There have long been concerns about appropriate referrals and the provision of sufficient information on discharge from hospital to district nursing teams within the community,[15,16] although perceptions of appropriateness can vary according to the primary or secondary setting. Pateman et al.[17] found that hospital nurses working in a cancer centre wanted to refer on most cancer patients to provide support for patients on discharge. District nurses interviewed within this study wanted early referral of palliative care patients to enable a firm basis of communication to be established but did not want patients to be referred purely as a check on progress after discharge. In part, the use of terminology such as supportive care may not have enabled precision in establishing referral need, and reaching a consensus on referral criteria may be difficult. Pateman et al. suggest that 'where a flexible, generic, holistic role is seen as desirable, inappropriate referrals may have to be accepted as the inevitable cost'.

### Multidisciplinary teamworking

Teamworking is an essential component part of palliative care and good collaborative relationships are important to enable effective communication of information. This is an area discussed repeatedly within other chapters. District nurses need to work across many teams including their own DN team, the primary healthcare team, the wider specialist palliative care team and teams involving social service colleagues. The differing working contexts, lack of understanding of each other's remits, and different perceptions of division of work and common goals can lead to a lack of continuity that can threaten good working relationships.[18,19]

Good channels of communication are essential to enable optimum patient care to be realised.[2] External pressures can affect the quality of these relationships. Such pressures include poor referral systems and overwork, as extensive caseloads can contribute to a lack of understanding of each other's roles, particularly where regular face-to-face meetings are not held.[2] Concerns over the changing nature of DN roles have been voiced over several years from the growth of social care to the increasing development of clinical nurse specialist posts.[20] Some specialist palliative care providers in Burt *et al.*'s study were concerned that overstressed DNs were sometimes not easy to contact and could sometimes leave CNSs to pick up community nursing work.

> There's no doubt about it that the services are pressurised. You know, when you've got – when you're carrying vacancies, year in and year out, then it means that everybody else is actually taking the pressure of that vacancy. And it's probably those pressures that mean that communication doesn't happen – they just haven't got the time to do it.
>
> (CNS)

From the DN perspective, however, there could be frustration at what was seen to be a departure from the time when CNSs provided hands-on care in the home to their role now of providing advice and support. When CNSs were in a patient's home, some DNs felt that they should provide nursing care, such as administering an enema, rather than call the DN out to do so. One DN commented on a CNS request for booking a Marie Curie nurse:

> And the instance of booking that Marie Curie nurse that time ... 'I've got the form here. I'll fax it to you and you can fill it in!' Why couldn't that person, knowing all the details of the particular patient, fill the form in and fax it off directly theirself ... as if we were the handmaids basically! It sounds very resentful, doesn't it? But I mean, you know, when we're all under pressure.
>
> (DN)

Good supportive relationships between the district nurse, GP and community specialist nurse were identified as essential to maintain the supportive triangle providing good continuity of care to patients. When one element of this triangle broke down, then care could be compromised.

Introduction of the Gold Standards Framework for Palliative Care (GSF) can improve teamworking both within the primary health-care team and with specialist palliative care services, and this is discussed further in Chapter 11. Use of the DN record held within the home can frequently provide continuity of information transfer. The DNs in one part of Scotland described how their patient-held records provide clear, accessible information for patients and carers, and list contact numbers for various personnel and services in hours and out of hours. They encourage GPs and Macmillan nurses to use their records (although not all GPs do so). This only applies, of course, to patients who are seeing the DN, which is more likely with those who are terminally ill.

In Scotland, professionals were generally very positive about out-of-hours communication, particularly between GPs and district nurses. Communication was enhanced where they were based in the same building. GPs often relied on district nurses to supplement information they received from daytime services. As one GP described:

> If we want to set up, say, a syringe-driver, the system is there to get that organised. The district nursing service, particularly for our co-op that we have is very good. They actually do provide a good deal of continuity because the district nurses that work for the co-op work during the day as well often and they know a lot of the patients in the local area who have got ongoing palliative care needs, so they can often inform us a great deal, give assistance regarding the current situation if perhaps the special notes aren't up to date.

A social worker described the challenges of teamworking in organising out-of-hours care:

> you might have problems with continuity of staff, because day staff and night staff might be very different, and for someone to be able to hit the ground running at half past nine or ten o'clock at night and have the trust of the patient, be confident about what they are doing, and you are working at kind of different stages of different

distances from one another, it's a very big challenge to get that right, so my issue is that the uncertainties and the unpredictability of people's conditions, make it hard for us to have enough time to plan things. And also that, for instance, if I am organising a care package and I liaise with my district nurse colleagues, they will do their utmost to link in with Marie Curie to try and get overnight cover.

Across England, the national education and support programme for district and community nurses in the principles and practice of palliative care improved communication and collaboration between services.[21] The programme provided Cancer Networks with additional resources to develop flexible local programmes focused around core areas such as symptom management and assessment. Initial proposals, submitted in 2001, were to provide evidence of collaboration with all educational providers and commissioners across a Network. In developing proposals and later implementing plans, collaborative working was established across Cancer Networks between specialist palliative care and hospice services and PCTs, and had spin-offs in terms of improved working relationships. DNs attending courses frequently provided by specialist colleagues developed better working relationships and knowledge about service remit and availability. The evaluation of this national initiative provides fuller details on how working relationships were improved.[21]

### Resource constraints

DN services, particularly in inner-city areas, can experience high recruitment and retention problems. Lack of staff and a resultant high use of agency staff can lead to a loss of morale as a result of excessive caseloads.[2] A national survey of community trusts undertaken in 1998 found that most did not have sufficient resources to deliver intermediate or acute nursing care at home.[22] Such under-resourcing has a clear impact on continuity of care. Over 10 years ago Seale identified concerns that DNs had that more could and should have been done for patients, particularly in terms of spending time with them and supporting families.[3] In the London study many DNs described how difficult it was to see palliative care patients alongside their usual caseload of patients with chronic problems.[2] Lack of time meant that they either had to severely restrict time taken with non-palliative patients, or not spend the time thought necessary with their palliative patients and families.

> You would like not to have to rush off; you would like to have to spend the time; you would like to do the little things that just make that person's life a little bit variable. And not for the person only – you've got to think of the whole family … and sometimes you just have to re-prioritise because you're just too short-staffed that you're then having to think: I know you need my care and I know you need my attention, but right now all I can do is just focus on that person that's in that bed right now. I'm going to have to run – and that's heartbreaking when you're having to drive away.

It is particularly within the out-of-hours period when resource constraints can bite and limited or no provision of a district nursing service result. In areas of high deprivation, such resource constraints can affect all services and any out-of-hours nursing cover be very difficult to provide.

### Out-of-hours care

The National Institute for Health and Clinical Excellence (NICE) Supportive and Palliative Care Guidance recommends that PCTs provide 24-hour DN services, and, where not, access for patients suffering from advanced cancer should be provided by other qualified nurses/care assistants.[23] DN service provision, however, is patchy particularly at night when many PCTs do not provide district nursing services. Dissatisfaction with the availability of DN out-of-hours services has been greater for night services than evening, which are more frequently available.[24] The audit commission investigated DN services in the latter part of the 1990s, and at that time one-third of community trusts had no DN night service.[15] A survey in 2004 found that similarly one-third of London PCTs still had no DN night service.[25] While many others provided day, twilight and night services, some did not provide these throughout 24 hours, with gaps in the early evening and early morning. Access to 24-hour community nursing services is a clear priority for DNs across London[2] but do present resource issues, as in many areas it is only safe for DNs to visit in pairs. In Scotland, out-of-hours nurses expressed concerns about their vulnerability, as they went out alone and appeared to have little faith in any alarm systems they had. In some areas, where the number of nurses on duty out of hours was small, visiting in pairs was not practical.[1]

In the Scottish study,[1] considerable variation in availability of district nurses out of hours was identified. Even within one Health Board, services could vary, with some dedicated evening and night services, other areas relying on daytime staff covering nights on a rota, and some areas having gaps in cover of an hour or two at certain times of the evening or night. Such variability was described by staff as a major factor in inequity of provision of services to palliative care patients out of hours:

> It just depends too much on where you live, what nursing service is available. We need a dedicated, rapid-response district nursing service for palliative care, and not just for people with cancer, so we have more time to spend with patients and families.
>
> (DN/palliative care nurse)

The difference between the level of service provision for palliative care patients by day and night was an issue:

> I think it is very, very important for the patients that there is conti-nuity of care. That they're not getting a certain standard during the day and they're getting a completely different standard at night.
>
> (Triage nurse)

Out-of-hours nursing provision was often described as under review, with a need for new service configurations to enable better responsiveness to patient and carer needs.

Despite these difficulties, there was much praise from palliative care patients and carers in the Scottish study who had access to dis-trict nurses. Some patients had regular visits from the nurses out of hours and found they gave better continuity of care than medi-cal services. One carer described how continuity enabled her to look after her husband at home during his terminal illness:

I think my husband liked the continuity of seeing the same person. He was a very quiet person and I think he liked to recognise the face and he was exceptionally ill at the end and then my mother had cancer and of course she liked continuity again as we older people do, and, I think, nobody thinks they are doing anything exceptional but I believe the fact that I, actually I, managed to keep my husband at home a lot of it was because I had continuity and I had great faith in the people that were behind me and I mean I really could not fault any of the services that my husband had. He had a kidney removed, it went into his bones, he had a brain tumour, lost his sight, he couldn't walk, you know but he was very, very ill but I think it was because I had such faith in the people that were about me were wonderful, that you know we managed it.[1]

Access to other nursing services out of hours has also been reported to be patchy. Marie Curie nursing services are important, particularly for the last days of life, but access can be limited.[2,9] Similarly, access to specialist palliative care services out of hours can be patchy and only just over 40 per cent of DNs were reported to be satisfied with their availability for advice and/or support out of hours.[9] DNs also report variable access to drugs out of hours across Cancer Networks, with just under one-third only reporting adequate access. In Scotland, the introduction of a community pharmacy model scheme for palliative care, with an on-call pharmacist available round the clock, was universally seen as having improved services, although there were some gaps in coverage.[1]

While there has been the introduction of nurse prescribing, out of hours many DNs remain dependent on the support of a GP, particularly for making medication changes. There have been concerns about access and the willingness of GPs to undertake home visits.[2]

**Opportunities to improve continuity of care**

The demand for DN night services has long been identified.[24,26] DNs and GPs in Burt et al.'s study were asked what services they would rate as priorities for future palliative care development.[2] Over 60 per cent of DNs and 41 per cent of GPs wanted to develop DN night services, although just under 40 per cent of DNs and only 20 per cent of GPs wanted to develop general medical services. Generally about 60 per cent of both professional groups preferred to develop specialist palliative care services such as access to in-patient beds, assessments, Macmillan nurses and, for DNs, Marie Curie nurses. Concern was greater amongst DNs for the provision of strengthened primary and nursing services to palliative care patients than amongst GPs.

The education and support programme for district and community nurses, funded by the Department of Health, has also presented opportunities for strengthening district nursing provision.[21] The key role that DNs play in palliative care has been confirmed by this programme and it has led to a first national assessment of the numbers of district nurses across the country, undertaken by Cancer Networks. While the aim was to establish educational needs, it also provided an opportunity to compare and contrast numbers of trained and untrained staff across the country with a view to establishing baseline standards of provision to enable good continuity in palliative care.

Funding sources that have emerged over the past few years to support development, particularly of specialist palliative care, have sometimes enabled the further development of DN services, mainly out of hours. An example is the New Opportunities funding provided by the Big Lottery Fund in 2003, which provided grants for the development of a range of services. These services were innovative, frequently addressing gaps in local provision, and supported better continuity of care through establishing multi-agency working between primary and community care services, and enabling access over 24 hours. Some examples of service developments funded are given in Table 4.1.

Finally, the development of the role of community matrons has the potential to enable greater coordination of care to be provided both within and out of hours. These posts present the opportunity for addressing some of the organisational issues that threaten collaboration between healthcare professionals. Palliative care is being established as a key component of the role within some PCTs. It will be important, however, that such roles are developed in partnership with GPs but not at the expense of removing skilled nurses from hands-on district nursing (palliative care) work.

Table 4.1 **Examples of schemes funded by the New Opportunities Fund**

| | |
|---|---|
| *St Wilfrids Hospice at Home Consortium, SE England* | The three-year scheme covers the Eastbourne Downs Primary Care Trust area to establish a joint Trust District Nursing and Hospice at Home service building on an earlier joint home care initiative, enabling terminally ill people to remain at home. It is supported by a broadly based multi-disciplinary team offering 24-hour care, coordinating existing services and adding complementary therapies and family support. Team members include nurses, care assistants, therapists and volunteers |
| *South Sefton PCT* | The 39-month scheme covers the South Sefton area in Liverpool. It employs nurses to provide 24-hour home-based palliative care and a social worker to support patients and carers with cancer and non-cancer conditions. The funding will also improve crisis and respite care, and access to out-of-hours support |
| *Derwentside out-of-hours palliative care nursing services* | An overnight community nursing service has been established for patients with palliative care needs over three years covering the Derwentside PCT area. A team of nurses deliver overnight home-based care for patients with palliative care needs, including cancer and other life-threatening conditions, particularly respiratory and neurological conditions |

## Conclusions

The district nursing service is an essential and central component in supportive and palliative care provided to patients and carers at home. As the service generally provides the most frequent number of visits and hands-on nursing care towards the end of life, coordinating the input of other services, in optimum circumstances it can provide personal continuity of care over time including informational, management and relational continuity as well as continuity of place as described at the outset. Pressured caseloads and skilled staffing shortages do pose a threat to continuity of care, as does the lack of a national 24-hour service. Multi-agency collaboration may well provide a way forward in better supporting palliative care patients and carers throughout 24 hours, but this requires continuing local effort in ensuring clarity over roles and good working relationships.

## Summary

- The provision of 24-hour district nursing services (or their equivalent) is a NICE priority and a development that many DNs would like to see introduced.

- Continuity of care out of hours requires good communication and working relationships between different professional groups within and out of hours. Early and appropriate referral to DN services enables the development of supportive relationships with patients and families.

- In terms of out-of-hours organisation of services, where community nursing services are based within a GP cooperative, then greater communication of information is possible together with joint visiting to better support patient care. Where services are not based together, bypass numbers to enable DNs to speak directly to the duty doctor improves the speed of communication.

- DN teams want greater access to 24-hour specialist support, Marie Curie and night-sitting services out of hours. Specialist provision is patchy in extent of service offered and geographical coverage. NICE guidance recommends that access to specialist telephone advice as a minimum should be mandatory. However, there is a need for evaluation of the varying range of specialist out-of-hours services to understand the different ways in which they can better support local primary healthcare professionals.

- Better access to other health and social services within and out of hours is essential to enable DNs to bring in additional help and resources when necessary. In providing and commissioning primary care services, PCTs need to reconsider the provision of GP home visits to palliative care patients out of hours to ensure availability and access at the time of need. Better access to palliative care drugs out of hours is an issue of concern.

**REFERENCES**

1. Worth A, Boyd K, Kendall M, Heaney D, Macleod U, Cormie P, Hockley J and Murray S. Out-of-hours palliative care: A qualitative study of cancer patients, carers and professionals. *British Journal of General Practitioners* 2006; **56 (522)**: 3–4.

2. Burt J, Shipman C, Addington-Hall J and White P. *Palliative Care. Perspectives on caring for dying people in London.* London: King's Fund, 2005.

3. Seale C. Community nurses and the care of the dying. *Social Science and Medicine* 1992; **34**: 375–82.

4. Goodman C, Knight D, Machen I and Hunt B. Emphasizing terminal care as district nursing work: A helpful strategy in a purchasing environment? *Journal of Advanced Nursing* 1998; **28**: 491–8.

5. Department of Health. *Making a Difference: Strengthening the nursing, midwifery and health visiting contribution to health and healthcare.* London: Department of Health, 1999.

6. CPHVA. *District Nursing at the Crossroads – A CPHVA briefing.* London: CPHVA, 2003.

7. Department of Health. *NHS Cancer Plan. Education and support for district and community nurses in the principles and practice of palliative care.* London: Department of Health, 2001.

8. Haggerty J L, Reid R J, Freeman G K, Starfield B H, Adair C E and McKendry R. Continuity of care: A multidisciplinary review. *British Medical Journal* 2003; **327 (7425)**: 1219–21.

9. Shipman C, Addington-Hall J, Richardson A, Burt J, Ream E and Beynon T. Palliative Care Services in England: a survey of district nurses' views. *British Journal of Community Nursing* 2005; **10**: 8, 381–6.

10. Grande G E, Farquhar C, Barclay S I G and Todd C J. Valued aspects of primary palliative care: Content analysis of bereaved carers' descriptions. *British Journal of General Practice* 2004; **54**: 772–8.

11. Fakhoury W, McCarthy M and Addington-Hall J. Determinants of informal caregivers' satisfaction with services for dying cancer patients. *Social Science and Medicine* 1996; **42 (5)**: 721–31.

12. Lecouturier J, Jacoby A, Bradshaw C, Lovel T and Eccles M. Lay carers' satisfaction with community palliative care: Results of a postal survey. South Tyneside MAAG Palliative Care Study Group. *Palliative Medicine* 1999; **13 (4)**: 275–83.

13. Hatcliffe S, Smith P and Daw R. District nurses' perceptions of palliative care at home. *Nursing Times* 1996; **92 (41)**: 36–7.

14. Wright K. Caring for the terminally ill: The district nurse's perspective. *British Journal of Nursing* 2002; **11**: 18, 1180–5.

15. Audit Commission. *First Assessment: A review of district nursing services in England and Wales.* London: Audit Commission Publications, 1999.

16. McKenna H, Keeney S and Nevin L. Perceptions of GPs and DNs on the role of hospice home-care nurses. *International Journal of Palliative Nursing* 1999; **15**: 288–95.

17. Pateman B, Wilson K, McHugh G and Luker K. Continuing care after cancer treatment. *Journal of Advanced Nursing* 2003; **44 (2)**: 192–9.

18. Bliss J and While A. Decision-making in palliative and continuing care in the community: An analysis of the published literature with reference to the context of UK care provision. *International Journal of Nursing Studies* 2003; **40**: 881–8.

19. Bliss J. District nurses' and social workers' understanding of each other's role. *British Journal of Community Nursing* 1998; 3; **7**: 330–6.

20. Luker K A, Wilson K, Pateman B and Beaver K. The role of district nursing: Perspectives of cancer patients and their carers before and after hospital discharge. *European Journal of Cancer Care* 2003; **12**: 308–16.

21. Addington-Hall J M, Shipman C, Burt J, *et al. Evaluation of the Education and Support Programme for District and Community Nurses in the Principles and Practice of Palliative Care. Report to the Department of Health*, 2006.

22. Edwards M and Dyson L. Is the district nursing service in a position to deliver intermediate care? A national survey of district nursing provision. *Primary Health Care Research and Development* 2003; **4**: 353–64.

23. National Institute for Clinical Excellence. *Guidance on Cancer Services: Improving supportive and palliative care for adults with cancer – the manual.* London: NICE, 2004.

24. Shipman C, Addington-Hall J, Barclay S, Briggs J, Cox I, Daniels L and Millar D. Providing palliative care in primary care: How satisfied are GPs and district nurses with current out-of-hours arrangements? *British Journal of General Practice* 2000; **50**: 477–8.

25. Shipman C, Addington-Hall J M, Richardson A, Burt J, Ream A and Beynon T. 24-hour district nursing services for palliative care patients: The challenge for cancer networks. Abstract in *Palliative Medicine* 2004; **18 (2)**: 368.

26. Barclay S, Todd C, McCabe J and Hunt T. The differing priorities of general practitioners and district nurses for palliative care services: Implications for commissioning by primary care groups. *British Journal of General Practice* 1999; **49**; 181–6.

CHAPTER | 5

# Patient and carer perspectives of continuity in palliative care

*Allison Worth and Dan Munday*

## Introduction

It is a fundamental principle of current healthcare policy that, in order to make services more acceptable, accessible and effective, patient and carer experiences and views must be understood and incorporated into service design.[1,2] At times of rapid and radical change in the delivery of primary care and out-of-hours services, it is important to assess patient and carer perspectives of services and the implications of new developments for their care.

This chapter will draw on two research studies that interviewed palliative care patients and their carers about their contact with out-of-hours and emergency services, giving unique and important insights into their experiences and their perspectives of their needs. One study was conducted in Scotland in 2001–3 and interviewed palliative care patients and their carers about their recent use of out-of-hours services.[3] The other was an interview study of patients with advanced illness admitted as emergencies to hospital beds in a large district general hospital in the English Midlands (2000–1).[4]

## Background

There are two main aspects to providing a comprehensive out-of-hours palliative care service. Patients sometimes need emergency care when deterioration occurs unexpectedly. Such care is largely provided by GPs and district nurses, with hospital and hospice admissions as a back-up. Palliative care patients and their carers also need supportive, pre-organised care out of hours to enable people to remain at home through provision of effective symptom management and carer support. Supportive and palliative care is essential to enable people to die at home if that is what they and their carers wish. These services are generally provided by general practitioners (GPs), district nurses, social care and sitting services from either statutory or voluntary agencies. Specialist palliative care back-up may be required in both emergency and supportive care.

Recent changes in services mean that patients are unlikely to see a doctor who knows them out of hours, making continuity of care problematic. They are also less likely to receive a home visit, with out-of-hours centres and telephone advice replacing the home as the locus of out-of-hours care.[5] Patients in general may regret the loss of the continuity of care associated with a more personal 24-hour GP service and retain expectations of a service based on home visiting.[5-7] For palliative care patients in particular, concerns have been expressed that the loss of continuity may contribute to unnecessary admission to hospital and reduce patient choice in place of death.[8] Current out-of-hours systems may therefore create conflict for practitioners in delivering the essential principles of palliative care.

There are undoubtedly challenges to incorporating patient views in end-of-life research and service development. Numerous barriers hinder the identification of the views of very ill patients: ethical, practical and recruitment problems abound.[9] Some studies have gathered the views of health professionals and carers about out-of-hours palliative care,[10,11] but few have directly gathered the views and experiences of palliative care patients themselves. Studies that have gathered carer views post-bereavement have identified both satisfaction and problems with end-of-life continuity of care.[12,13] Carers' perceptions and recall of events, however, may differ from the patient's experience.

**Study A: palliative care out of hours: patient and carer views**

The Scottish study[3] was conducted in three contrasting areas, urban, semi-urban and rural, reflecting the national diversity of settings for out-of-hours service delivery. The study gathered the views of palliative care cancer patients and their informal carers about their needs and their experiences of services out of hours. We explored with patients and their carers how they made the decision whether or not to contact out-of-hours services as well as their experiences of receiving care. Interviews took place between 2001 and 2003, just prior to the introduction of NHS24. (NHS24 is the Scottish equivalent of NHS Direct. It was introduced gradually between 2002 and 2004. It now provides a single point of access to out-of-hours services across Scotland.)

In-depth interviews were conducted with 32 patients with advanced cancer and 19 carers. Most interviews took place in the patient's or carer's home. Those included were patients with a diagnosis of advanced cancer who were receiving palliative treatment (palliative chemotherapy or radiotherapy) or care (supportive and terminal care), and who had recently used the out-of-hours service. Eight focus groups comprising 55 people were also conducted, in order to gain a broader perspective, from users and non-users, of their views of out-of-hours services. Focus group participants were recruited through a day hospice, a hospital-based cancer services user group, a hospice carers' group and through carer involvement workers. This allowed us to capture a range of views, including from people with cancer who had used the out-of-hours service and those who had not, and bereaved carers. Interviews and focus groups were tape recorded and data were analysed using constant comparative method, with the aid of NVivo software.

### Why did palliative care patients and their carers call the out-of-hours service?

The most common reason given for calling the out-of-hours service was pain, sometimes sudden and severe, and sometimes, particularly for patients at the end of life, poorly controlled. The next most common reason was nausea or vomiting, sometimes associated with chemotherapy. A variety of other reasons were given for contacting out-of-hours services, including bleeding, breathlessness, raised temperature, confusion, falls and various less specific symptoms, such as shaking, weakness or a 'funny turn'. Occasionally, urgent support needs, such as the carer being taken ill, prompted the call.

This focus on physical needs, however, disguises a more complex picture. When telephoning the out-of-hours service, patients and carers perhaps emphasised the physical symptoms in order to establish their legitimacy as in need of urgent attention. When describing the reasons for contacting the out-of-hours service to the researcher, patients and carers often talked about the fear and anxiety they experienced. This was often connected to uncertainty about the meaning of the physical symptoms: did sudden onset of pain or physical or mental deterioration indicate a relapse, or the onset of the terminal phase of the illness, or would it resolve without intervention?

Patients and carers also acknowledged that problems often appear magnified at night:

> It's usually at night that I've needed the service, and I know that's probably a bad thing on my part, but everything seems to be worse at night.
>
> (Patient C)

> Most people's emergencies do happen out of hours. In the middle of the night when you feel totally alone and abandoned.
>
> (Carer, focus group)

### What barriers did patients and carers face in contacting out-of-hours services?

An array of difficulties emerged for patients and carers who sought help out of hours. Some related to their own uncertainties about their needs and the services available. Other difficulties appeared more related to an out-of-hours service that was not designed to meet the needs of palliative care patients (see Box 5.1).

### Patients' and carers' own uncertainties about their needs

Most patients and carers struggled to make the decision to call the out-of-hours service. The main factors that contributed to this difficulty were:

---

Box 5.1 **Factors inhibiting patients and carers from contacting out-of-hours services**

---

- Uncertainty about the severity of their condition and urgency of their needs.
- Fear of being a nuisance and 'bothering the doctor'.
- Not knowing what was wrong or being unable to describe the problem clearly.
- Experience of daytime services; difficulty getting appointments.
- Not knowing who to call.
- Low expectations of out-of-hours services.
- Having to speak to someone who does not know you.
- Out-of-hours services lacking information on the patient's specific needs and history.
- Perceptions of triage as hostile.
- Fear of hospital admission.
- Previous bad experiences.

---

### *Judging whether their condition was severe enough and urgent enough to warrant calling an out-of-hours service*

Patients and carers often worried about whether professionals would view them as legitimate users of the out-of-hours service. They did not want to ask for help unnecessarily and feared being labelled a nuisance or that sanctions might be taken against them if they called the doctor without good reason. This appeared to reflect deep-seated cultural beliefs, particularly among older people: patients and carers talked of being brought up not to 'bother the doctor' and of a sense of responsibility to be a good patient, not calling the doctor out of hours unless absolutely necessary. One woman explained how she felt about having to call the out-of-hours service:

> I've been lucky I've not had to do it that often, but now I'm having to do it, I feel it's difficult you know, more so because you feel as though you are being a bit of a nuisance, and even being so ill I still feel 'oh no, I'll have to phone them' you know. I still go through that. My sisters blame my mum 'cos my mum would never call out a doctor unless you are absolutely in your bed dying.
>
> (Patient G)

A carer talked about how she delayed contacting the out-of-hours service:

> you wait until it's so horrendous until you think 'I canna cope any more, I need somebody else to come in here and make a decision, is there anywhere I can go, is there anybody that can help me, could you?
>
> (Carer, focus group)

Patient and carer experiences of access to services in the daytime also appeared to affect and influence their decisions out of hours. A frequent theme in the focus groups was the difficulty of obtaining a GP appointment or a home visit and the number of questions the receptionist asks. Patients and carers often perceived the out-of-hours service, and GPs in particular, as very busy. Some also worried that others might have greater need and that they might therefore be preventing someone else from getting the service. These factors led to patients and carers often exploring a variety of sources of out-of-hours help and advice first: friends, family, knowledgeable neighbours, and hospital or hospice staff were all mentioned by patients and carers as prompting them to call the out-of-hours service. It appeared to help them to overcome some of their anxieties about phoning for help if someone else told them they should:

> I was very fortunate I had a nursing sister that stays next door to me and the day that my husband died I knew things were not right at all and I asked her to come in and she just said 'you phone the hospice right now' and so I mean somebody else really sort of prompted me to do it because I didn't know.
>
> (Carer, focus group)

### Not knowing what was wrong or lacking the appropriate language to describe it

Carers talked of the difficulties they faced in caring for someone who is terminally ill, how they often feel isolated and ill-prepared to deal with symptoms that occurred unexpectedly, not knowing what to do and feeling cut off from their usual daytime support systems. All these factors contributed to the difficulty of making decisions, as two carers in a focus group indicated:

Carer A: 'I think at the last stages of an illness it's not just the patient but their carer. I wasn't in my right mind'

Carer B: 'You're not thinking straight, you need a professional to guide you.'

Some suggested that they needed someone to phone for advice and reassurance out of hours:

Carer C: 'I think if you had some [one to phone], particularly out of hours, because that's when it's really scary. You are not necessarily needing a doctor to come out but just somebody.'

Carer D: 'Yeah, somebody to talk to, like if it's just the pain, or it's just somebody's having hallucinations or sweats or things like that, because when these things happen the first time you don't know, nobody tells you "oh he's going to have these sweats" and nobody tells you how to cope, so if you could phone up.'

This suggests that a telephone service can provide useful support, as long as patients and carers can talk to someone knowledgeable about palliative care and with time to listen and give advice, preferably with information about that particular patient.

### Not knowing who to call or what to expect

Patients and carers who had not previously used the out-of-hours system had little knowledge of what services were available or how to obtain help. Some had no contact numbers, but, even if they did, could find the system confusing:

We had all the numbers, but weren't really always sure quite who was who. It can be a bit overwhelming at first.

(Patient B)

Some patients and carers had low expectations of the out-of-hours service, based on media reports, hearsay or other people's experiences, and this could add to their reluctance to phone the service for the first time. Some were pleasantly surprised when they did so:

The very first time that we used them we really thought 'och, they're going to send somebody out here that's going to just be unbelievable' because [of] everything that I thought about people doing these as extra services … it's extra money, that's what it's all about at the end of the day and I thought we were really going to end up with someone who perhaps was just qualified, or whatever, who had difficulty with the English language. All sorts of things that were really going to be going over their head and, contrary to that experience it wasn't, it was absolutely wonderful!

(Patient L)

Others suggested that their low expectations were realised:

That's the first time I've ever had to deal wi' them but it'll be the last. I won't bother again.

(Carer, focus group)

Another blamed herself for the GP not providing a home visit out of hours:

I was blaming myself thinking I was going about it the wrong way you know, I wisnae [i.e. was not] asking the right questions, I wisnae saying the right things to get them to come and have a look at him.

(Carer, focus group)

Occasionally, patients and carers preferred the idea of contacting out-of-hours services rather than their own GP, as they knew they were not getting someone out of bed to attend to them. Two carers in a focus group said:

Carer E: 'quite honestly I think I would phone the out of hours, luckily it hasn't happened too often, I'd feel more comfortable phoning the out of hours than phoning up my own GP at night.'

Carer F: 'Oh definitely, because you know the out of hours is always there.'

A patient said:

You feel so reassured you know that there's somebody there, willing to help you straight away, or as soon as they possibly can.

(Patient B)

### Concerns about lack of continuity of care

Continuity of care is important to people with palliative care needs and their carers, and this is something the out-of-hours service does not normally offer. Many patients and carers recognised that it is not feasible for their own GPs and specialist staff to be available around the clock. It did appear, however, to be a contributory factor in patients' and carers' reluctance to contact out-of-hours services. Uncertainty about the response and having to see a GP or nurse who did not know you were often barriers to seeking help. As one carer said:

> You see I would have done anything but phone the out of hours. If I could have phoned our own nurses I wouldn't have thought anything about it. Because you know who you're speaking [to]. If it was our own doctors I would know because I mean they're just like friends, as far as I am concerned, but it's this business, you don't know what you're going to get at the other end.
>
> (Carer J)

A patient said:

> it's just part of impersonalisation of everything and you're just a number.
>
> (Patient L)

One patient, who had used the out-of-hours service on a number of occasions, described his lack of confidence in a system that does not provide continuity of care:

> the doctor who does come out, not only does he not have any notes about me, but he doesn't know me at all. As a person, he doesn't know me but he spends time trying to get to know me before he can think about my condition. It doesn't help my confidence in him. I've got to decide does this doctor know what he's doing you know? So that is a problem.
>
> (Patient I)

His wife highlighted the problems associated with trying to understand the complex history of palliative care patients without the relevant information and knowledge:

> I do think an out-of-hours service, the doctors are very handi-

capped in a number of situations and particularly say 'I am a doctor but I'm not your GP and I don't really know you know, all that's been going on.'

(Carer I)

Some patients and carers had been encouraged to contact the hospital or hospice rather than out-of-hours services and perceived this as providing greater continuity of care:

> I personally found that at the hospital we were always told if you have a problem phone us. I mean if I was stuck I would have phoned my GP, just 'cos we got on very well with him but I knew that either the hospital or the hospice nurse, they had far more information than my GP had.

(Carer, focus group)

Some patients and carers, however, said they would call an ambulance rather than try to seek help via the out-of-hours service. One patient, who felt his needs had not been met by the out-of-hours service, said:

> If something drastic had happened here that night, I would have ended up being collected in a box … it has really put me off phoning them. … I feel safer with the hospital … I feel I would just get in or get an ambulance, bypass the out of hours.

(Patient A)

When the GP or nurse who saw the patient displayed knowledge and competence, instilled confidence and gave information, it could help to override patients' and carers' anxieties about lack of continuity:

> I think when you're ill you're just grateful that someone is seeing to you. It would be wonderful if it was your own doctor but realistically how could your own doctor possibly ever give that sort of service? They just couldn't. So, no, as long as someone comes out who's competent, who does what's necessary then no, I don't think it matters at all that it's not your own doctor, in an ideal world of course it would be lovely but if they're seeing me at 8 o'clock at night they're certainly not going to see me in a normal appointment next morning so it can't work for them.

(Patient L)

## Information

Another aspect of continuity of care that often concerns health professionals is the lack of information available to out-of-hours personnel. Patients and carers also showed awareness of this problem:

> at the out-of-hours centre they don't have access to that patient's files, so they don't know the patient's circumstances.
>
> (Carer, focus group)

> he couldn't really make sort of major decisions and that I think is a major issue because they don't know, it's always a stranger. ... I do think an out-of-hours service, the doctors are very handicapped in a number of situations and particularly ours, if they don't have access to records.
>
> (Carer I)

Some patients reported positively on out-of-hours services that knew about them already, their own GP having passed information on.

## Patients and carers perceived various service barriers

Patients and carers often felt that the process of accessing out-of-hours services presented a further difficulty. The triage system was the focus of their concerns, poorly understood by many patients and carers, who saw it as presenting a barrier to the generally desired outcome of their call, a home visit.

Some patients and carers perceived the routine questions they were asked as part of the triage process as hostile:

> First of all it's like 'Do you really need this service? Is it an emergency?' And you think well aye, I suppose it is. You don't know whether you should phone or not or just ride the storm out and that's wrong because, obviously if you're feeling anxious enough to be phoning a GP in the first place, there is a cause and they should be coming out ... they should trust your assessment of the situation.
>
> (Carer, focus group)

Having to repeat the same information to a number of staff was also perceived as a problem:

You speak to a receptionist, you tell her everything that's wrong and she says 'Hold on and I'll put you through to the nurse'. You have to tell the nurse again and then 'I'll go and speak to the doctor and get the doctor to phone you back'.

(Carer, focus group)

Patients and carers were often asked to attend the out-of-hours centre and many described feeling guilty for being unable to do so:

she says to me 'Would I make it down, could I make it down myself' and I said 'no', I said 'I am really sorry there is no way', more so because I don't get out and about myself because I've got advanced cancer if that's what you call it, it's breast cancer but it's spread, so I don't get out and about myself anyway. It's when you're asked though if you could make it down it makes you feel 'oh no', 'cos you've got to say 'no' you know. Even if they brought out transport but there would have been no way on the last two occasions, no way could I have got myself up and dressed and got down there.

(Patient G)

A minority of patients and carers expressed a positive view of triage:

I've found the response very good, the person who takes the call is very calm and asks you the minimum of questions and then the doctor rings you back and he has a discussion and then he either comes or initially when Mr I was well enough, we went down to the hospital.

(Patient I)

Other barriers to continuity of care out of hours, such as lack of time and resources, well known to professionals, seemed less apparent to patients and carers, who rarely mentioned them.

### What were patients' and carers' views of the service responses they received out of hours?

The majority of patients and carers perceived a home visit as the most appropriate response to their call to the out-of-hours service. Some bereaved carers reported good experiences of out-of-hours services, with staff who responded kindly, provided a home visit and who had time to attend to their needs:

> My personal experience of the out of hours was when I nursed my husband at home, he died of cancer just about, not quite, two years ago and he fell out of bed during the night and the cancer was on his back, everywhere really and I phoned and I got this wonderful young lady doctor and she came out at three in the morning and I just couldn't fault her, she was just amazing.
>
> (Carer, focus group)

> we had the evening nurses who were great, and they just came in for half an hour and you know instead of us hoisting my sister up, they took charge of that because it was all quite nerve wracking when you're not used to doing that kind of thing.
>
> (Carer, focus group)

> I had a night service. … I was offered it and I said no I was coping and then I had them two nights the last week, the night before he died and two nights before and they were absolutely brilliant.
>
> (Carer, focus group)

Although most patients preferred a home visit, carers occasionally reported being satisfied with telephone advice, particularly if the GP offered follow-up if the situation did not resolve:

> I phoned up the out-of-hours centre, and it was a lady doctor, and I told her what was wrong, and she gave me instructions over the phone, and then she told me that if everything, if he wisnae all right by the morning, she would fax my own doctor and I had to tell and phone them as well and they would come and see me.
>
> (Carer, focus group)

One woman who had often used the out-of-hours service said that both the severity of her condition and being known to the service were important influences on her care:

> we've been really very pleased with the service here, I've had no difficulties as such. Any time I call them they've been really happy to come out … they've been lovely, when they've came out they've been so thorough. … On the times that I've went to visit the centre, it's always been really quick, I've never had to wait very long. … I

did feel that having the illness I had, which was lymphoma, you seem to get the service there and then. There was no questions asked, it was just, yes you need the service, we're there.

(Patient H)

Good communication made the world of difference to patients' and carers' experiences of out-of-hours care. When patients and carers were told by the visiting GP or nurse what to expect, what signs to look for, what to do if certain things happen, and were given permission to phone again, this helped to allay their anxieties and gave them confidence about coping:

My friend was with me the first time and she said that she felt very confident of them because they not only spoke to me, but they then came and explained to her what was happening, what to expect in the next few hours and also to be on the lookout for certain things within the next few hours, so she felt aware of the situation and would have been able to respond accordingly.

(Patient L)

A carer described how good communication could defuse patients' and carers' worries:

he was so very nice to my dad and put him at ease and sat and listened to his story, father went through it all again … he had a delightful bedside manner, he was very nice indeed, also did not give the impression as so many doctors do, that he was in a hurry. … in fact he was here half an hour which was wonderful. … He examined him and was very kind to him, gave him an injection, father settled, father was absolutely delighted with the treatment and went off to sleep and woke up a different man, he was fine.

(Carer D)

Unfortunately, poor service responses were also identified. Patients and carers who had bad experiences of the out-of-hours service were put off contacting them again:

on the last two days before he died he was at home, and he was in the most dreadful pain at 7 o'clock at night, roaring with pain and I phoned the out of hours and I asked could I give him more morphine and the doctor said 'no, he's had enough, it will work eventually', so after two hours he did eventually fall asleep but this put me off from phoning again and, of course, he woke in the middle of the night and he was hallucinating, as they sometimes do with morphine, he was particularly bad for that, and I should have phoned the out of hours again but that small incident just kind of put me off phoning back.

(Carer, focus group)

Sometimes, a home visit did not produce a satisfactory outcome, as one patient recalled:

the one who was so unhelpful just wrote out a prescription – this was at 7 p.m. on a Sunday night. He waved it in the air and said, 'I don't know where you'll get this at this time of day' and went! Not helpful!

(Patient B)

## Do patients and carers worry about out-of-hours admissions?

Professionals have expressed concern that the lack of continuity of care out of hours leads to inappropriate admissions to hospital.[14] Some patients and carers shared this concern, linking it to GPs' perceptions of risk.

A carer said:

that's the other concern I have when it's a strange doctor and they will not want to take risks, neither of us really want Mr I booked into hospital, you know, and our own doctor understands that and is very supportive but if you've called someone out in the night you are dependent on how they assess the situation and you really don't know. If you say 'No, he's not going to hospital' you don't really know whether he has a really valid reason.

(Carer I)

Although most patients and carers were anxious to remain at home if possible, admission was sometimes welcomed if symptoms were severe or frightening. Among the patients in the study who were admitted to hospital as a consequence of their call to the out-of-hours service, none described it as inappropriate, even if they came home the next day.

### Discussion

The study highlights the problems experienced out of hours by people with advanced cancer at the end of life and their carers. The out-of-hours system has been set up to manage all demand for 24-hour care more effectively, but may not meet the special needs of palliative care patients. Patients and carers often do not know how to manage unexpected deterioration and lack effective support to enable them to cope with the physical and emotional demands of end-of-life care.

We spoke to many satisfied patients and carers, and identified good practice and a real commitment on the part of many key professionals to deliver good palliative care around the clock. When the system fails to meet patients' and carers' needs, however, as we also found to various degrees, the experience can be deeply distressing. Many problems could be mitigated by better planning and provision of information by in-hours staff, but unpredictable needs will always occur at times. Continuity of care is greatly enhanced by good communication and provision of information, both between health professionals and patients and carers, and between different professionals and services.[15]

### Study B: emergency admissions of palliative care patients

The second study under consideration was conducted in a large district general hospital in the English Midlands in 2000–1. This was undertaken following an audit of patients' symptom control needs after emergency admission. An unexpected finding of the audit was that 50 per cent of the patients admitted were following a 999 call rather than as a result of GP contact. The study aims were to explore the reasons for admission and the route taken into hospital.

Patients with palliative care needs, defined as 'non curable malignant disease in an advanced stage, who may or may not have been receiving palliative radio or chemotherapy', or patients with 'advanced life-threatening non malignant disease' were identified over five sample weeks from hospital admission data. Of the 81 patients identified, 30 were recruited whilst on the hospital wards if they were considered well enough to be approached and agreed to being interviewed. A further seven interviews were undertaken with relatives, either because the patient requested this or the relative of a patient who was judged too unwell was available and willing to be interviewed.

Interviews explored the reason for the patient's admission, who the patient called and reasons for selecting that particular professional or service. Patients were interviewed within three days of admission, to enable the narrative to emerge as close as possible to the event, which had not been modified by time and reflection. The interviews were relatively brief – 10–20 minutes and were recorded manually. This was a necessary compromise since patients were interviewed normally by their bedsides and many were easily tired. A striking finding was how keen patients were to share their story with the interviewer. The interview transcripts were analysed for emerging themes and coded using NVivo.

Patients in this study were not necessarily admitted out of hours; however, hospital admission in itself represents a break in continuity of place (see Chapter 1) as the patient moves from community to hospital care. Results do illustrate the ways in which patients may attempt to maintain continuity and control.

Similar themes to the Scottish study emerged, particularly the patients' views of some of the barriers faced accessing in- and out-of-hours GP services, difficulty in knowing when to call and some poor experiences of contact with services. Since the primary aim of the study was to capture patients' narratives about what had happened leading to the current admission, it is the themes emerging from these narratives that are presented here.

**Reasons for admission**

As in the Scottish study, many of the patients were admitted with uncontrolled symptoms, principally pain, nausea and vomiting, breathlessness and weakness. Patients with non-malignant disease were more likely to have been admitted with breathlessness. Patients would describe symptoms frequently in the context of the wider effect of the symptom. The patient below described how her symptoms had affected her ability to function as a mother and wife, and the feelings of guilt associated. (The following 'quotes' are paraphrases of interviews taken from field note manual recordings of interviews.)

Her problems were that she was feeling increasingly weak. She has no appetite and couldn't be bothered to eat. She also could only get up and downstairs on her hands and knees. In the time since she had been unwell over the last two weeks, her husband had to do increasing amounts at home. ... She feels that her husband is left to do everything and the children (13 and 15) don't help. This makes her feel quite guilty as he has to do these things when he comes back from work. She feels guilty about not being able to do simple things such as reaching for the telephone from the bed and having to call him to get it for her. She said some days things were better than other days and she just couldn't tell how she was going to be. For instance on some days she had still been able to cook.

(Patient 12 – woman with cancer)

Other patients were admitted with complications of their disease, such as spinal cord compression or haemoptysis. A further group of patients were admitted with complications of palliative treatments such as swallowing difficulties following radiotherapy to the upper respiratory tract or neutropenic sepsis following chemotherapy. Occasionally patients were admitted because of collapse or a rapidly deteriorating condition.

He always feels breathless and is on constant oxygen. He is only able to get to the toilet with help and get dressed with help from his wife. He was sitting on the toilet on Saturday afternoon when he collapsed. He does not know what happened. The first thing he knows is that he was lying on the ground. His neighbours had come over to help his wife. He might have been unconscious for around about five minutes.

(Patient 75 – man with end-stage fibrosing alveolitis)

Table 5.1 **Route of admission**

| Mode of Admission | Malignant | Non-malignant |
|---|---|---|
| GP – emergency admissions (EAU) | 18 (35%) | 13 (44%) |
| Patient/carer – 999 | 7 (13%) | 15 (52%) |
| From out-patient clinic | 6 (12%) | 1 (4%) |

| | | |
|---|---|---|
| Patient/carer – oncology ward | 7 (13%) | |
| GP – consultant oncologist | 3 (6%) | |
| Specialist nurse – oncologist | 2 (4%) | |
| Palliative care domiciliary visit | 2 (4%) | |
| District nurse – 999 | 2 (4%) | |
| GP – oncology ward | 1 (2%) | |
| Patient/carer – EAU | 1 (2%) | |
| Patient/carer – consultant oncologist | 1 (2%) | |
| Not specified | 2 (4%) | |
| **Total** | **52 (100%)** | **29 (100%)** |

Routes of admission for patients with malignant disease differed from patients with non-malignant disease, in that the cancer patients were admitted by many different routes. Table 5.1 describes the routes of admission for all 81 patients identified. The normal mode of admission for patients to this hospital is via the Emergency Admissions Unit (EAU) whether they are brought in by ambulance or referred by their GP. In this setting they are triaged and either admitted to a general ward, oncology ward if beds are available or discharged home if that is judged appropriate. Patients with cancer and under the care of an oncologist may be admitted directly onto the oncology ward mostly at the discretion of the nurse in charge. This may be at the request of a GP but more usually it is following a call directly from the patient to the ward. This system is designed to allow rapid admission of patients with neutropenic sepsis to the oncology ward but was actually used more generally for symptom control or other crisis admission. Patients often develop a close relationship with the oncology ward and there was evidence that patients might even use the oncology ward as a primary source of advice and care.

He cannot praise the … oncology ward highly enough. He says that 'you can telephone them day or night for advice and they are always ready to help and are very pleasant'.

(Patient 36 – man with cancer)

**Who patients and their carers called**

The choice patients and their carers make about whom to call in which situation seems to be influenced most clearly by three factors.

### *The professionals with whom the patient has an ongoing relationship*

Patients often indicated that their GP was rather distant from their care, often having not seen them for several months. This was true for patients with both malignant and non-malignant disease.

> He has been in hospital twice in the last six months both for between five and 10 days. He has not seen his GP for about six months. He finds it difficult getting out of the house to see him although last time the GP did come to see him at home when he was called.
>
> (Patient 74 – man with COPD)

> She has not seen her GP for about three months, when her GP paid a courtesy visit after the diagnosis of her cancer. She says 'there has been no point in seeing my GP as I get my medication on repeat prescription'. She goes on to say 'not sure what the GP could do for me – in any case her surgery is on the first floor and with breathing like mine it is very difficult to get up the stairs'.
>
> (Patient 37 – woman with cancer)

In contrast district nurses often took a central role in monitoring the patient's condition and providing advice and solutions when problems are faced.

> The district nurse calls every other week if she is asked and phones up every now and again to check on how she is.
>
> (Patient 69 – man with cancer)

The district nurse was often therefore the professional who was first involved in assisting the patient in a crisis situation, either by the patient waiting for her appointed visit, or by the patient or carer calling for advice.

> The district nurse had come out to him on the Tuesday and they had discussed how he felt. She said it would take longer for him to

get things sorted out if he went through the GP as he was going to the day centre the next day (Wednesday). 'Obviously it did because I saw the district nurse on the Tuesday and was admitted on the Thursday which was very quick.'

(Patient 69 – man with cancer)

However, patients with non-malignant diseases were less likely to have district nurse involvement in their care on a regular basis. This may be related to the fact that district nurses increasingly are only involved in task-based activities, such as wound care, setting up syringe drivers, etc. Patients with non-malignant diseases are probably less likely to need specific nursing tasks to be performed than cancer patients, and therefore less likely to have district nurses 'checking up' to make sure all is well.

District nurses were involved in contacting GPs who then admitted the patient to hospital.

As she had deteriorated the district nurses were visiting more regularly. On Sunday morning they came in to see her spontaneously having visited the day before. They telephoned the doctor themselves. A 'health call' doctor came to see her and suggested admission.

(Patient 31 – woman with cancer)

Other professionals such as palliative care nurse specialists and specialists in palliative medicine were involved in the care of some of the patients in the study and occasionally were involved in the admission process. Specialist nurses and GPs had access to consultant oncologists, with whom they liaised for patient admissions. No patient with non-malignant disease mentioned the involvement of a specialist nurse in the community.

Since patients with non-malignant disease had few other health professionals involved, their lack of contact with GPs on a regular basis gave the impression of a marked isolation from healthcare services in the community.

### The service or professional who the patient judged as being available

Patients and their carers made a judgement about who was available at what time and would choose who to call in an emergency situation partly on the grounds of this perceived availability. This meant that if they felt a service may be slow in responding they would seek help from an alternative.

District nurses as well as visiting regularly and maintaining a relationship with the patients were also seen as being accessible, either directly:

> The district nurses were visiting twice a week and coming straight away at other times if called.
>
> (Patient 12 – woman with cancer)

or for telephone advice in helping the patient to know what to do next:

> She phoned the district nurse who said it was better if they contacted the oncology ward as it was the weekend.
>
> (Patient 30 – woman with cancer)

This contrasted with GPs who were often seen as being less accessible, especially out of hours, as this same patient reported:

> They have waited up to 4 hours for a GP to call at the weekend and think it is a waste of time to call them. 'The GPs ask you to tell you them your history from the beginning and then they tell you to go to hospital anyway.'

The oncology ward again was seen as being available 24 hours per day, seven days per week. Following her contact with the district nurse, the same patient was admitted to the ward. She clearly feels reassured and safe on the oncology ward, which she contrasts to the general hospital wards.

> The oncology doctors have also told her to telephone the oncology ward for any problem whatsoever. She thinks this is very good, but the problem arises when there are no beds on the oncology ward. She then has to go to the general hospital which she describes as 'hell on earth'.

This stark expression needs to be understood in context. The busyness and lack of continuity (as it is likely a patient will go to a different ward for each admission), in comparison to the personal nature of the smaller oncology wards, may well be at least as important as any sense of inferior care being given on general hospital wards.

Patients with non-malignant diagnoses had two possible routes to admission: one via the GP; and the more common route into hospital that seemed to be through the ambulance service with the patient or informal carer dialling 999. As we have seen, some patients felt that hospital admission was inevitable and at times preferable to remaining in the community. In addition, some patients did contrast the rapid response of the ambulance service in comparison with the slowness of response from general practitioners.

> At about 5 p.m. I could take no more. My wife called the GP but the GP was not in. She was out seeing another patient. The receptionist told my wife to call for an ambulance and I also told her to dial 999. The ambulance came in about three minutes, they were very quick. They are always very quick.
>
> (Patient 59 – man with COPD)

The practice of calling for an ambulance to enable immediate admission was also reinforced by health professionals, including ambulance crews and hospital staff.

> When he called the ambulance last year the crew told him that in a similar situation in the future he should call them directly rather than anyone else, 'because we are the only ones who can help you'.
>
> (Patient 1 – man with COPD)

> She was advised by somebody (she thinks at the hospital) to call an ambulance rather than a GP if she needs to come in. She feels that the GP takes too long to come, it might be several hours.
>
> (Patient 13 – woman with COPD)

Also calling for an ambulance could be reinforced by the practice of primary care teams or GPs.

> On Tuesday morning his wife went out and when she came back he was very short of breath and getting rather panicky. She decided that she would not call for an ambulance and paramedic at that point but phoned the GP surgery for a home visit. 'They all know about his problems at the surgery and I talked to one of the recep-

tionists. Dr A said to the receptionist that he would arrange to get him admitted.' Dr A organised the ambulance.

(Patient 48 – man with cancer)

Clearly situations exist in which a call for an ambulance for immediate admission is entirely appropriate, for example in cases of unexpected collapse or severe central chest pain, since delay in admission and treatment may affect outcome adversely. However, it is possible that lack of clinical assessment may lead to the admission of patients who could have been clinically managed at home. Therefore it could be argued that for palliative care patients prompt attention from a medical practitioner in the community should be the norm.

### The professional or service in whom the patient felt confidence to deal with this situation effectively

All patients in this study were presented with at least two services that could be called in the emergency situation: their general practitioner, or out-of-hours GP services and the ambulance service. In addition, many had access to district nurses, and patients with malignant disease had several other possible courses of action, including telephoning directly to the oncology ward.

In making a choice about who it is appropriate to call, the patient weighs up not just the availability but also likelihood of an acceptable outcome. Some patients actively sought to come into hospital, often because they saw it as a place of safety and a place that could appropriately manage their condition.

He thinks in this situation it is always better to call the ambulance rather than the GP. Because 'he will only give you a couple of pills and leave you at home'.

(Patient 1 – man with COPD)

Occasionally she has been sent home from admissions but she feels more confident with this than with seeing her GP when she feels very ill.

(Patient 13 – woman with COPD)

On the morning of admission he asked his partner to call the ambulance as he was very breathless and was unable to move.

(Patient 23 – man with lung cancer)

For cancer patients this would often lead to directly calling the ward or returning directly to it.

> She was discharged four days before her readmission this time as they wanted to take her home for a break. However, she was in such pain that she asked her daughter to take her back to oncology. Her husband phoned the oncology ward to tell them that she was on the way back in her daughter's car.
>
> (Patient 38 – woman with lung cancer)

In a parallel to the Scottish study, being acquainted with a knowledgeable person sometimes influenced the process of admission. In the following situation the patient was related to a senior nurse in the oncology unit. This is her account (as the carer) of the process that led to his admission:

> She went out to visit him because she'd heard that he was not very well. When she saw his condition she decided that he ought to be admitted. She phoned the ward to find out if there was a bed and as there was she arranged for him to be admitted.
>
> (Patient 55 – man with cancer)

## Discussion

This study is concerned with patients who had been admitted as emergencies into hospital beds. No patient in the study questioned the appropriateness of their admission. This is interesting since it is a major concern of strategists in palliative care and was certainly highlighted by participants in the Scottish out-of-hours study. Whilst it is regarded that advance care planning, availability of community services able to meet patients' need and 24-hour availability of experienced practitioners with information regarding the patient might enable patients to remain in their homes, it was not possible in this study to judge on this aspect. All patients interviewed had clearly consented to their admission and many had actively sought to be admitted to hospital. However, with clear lack of availability of some services in the community, patients often seemed to have little option than to be admitted to hospital.

**Concluding remarks**

Patients' and carers' experiences of accessing services in an urgent or emergency situation captured in both of these studies seem to be highly varied. Many experiences, however, illustrate how at present services can often be lacking and poorly coordinated, but how also individual practitioners are delivering care that is appreciated by patients and carers. It is important to be somewhat guarded about judging services on the experiences of patients and carers alone, since this only examines the issues from one perspective. At Warwick Medical School a study to examine emergency palliative care incidents from the multiple perspectives of patient, carer and healthcare professionals is underway. We hope to be able to capture some of the complexities of these situations in greater depth, allowing a fuller understanding of the issues.

A danger of the current debate around 'preferred place of death' is that it could fail to recognise the complexity of palliative care in the community. Whilst patient choice of place of care and death is important, and few patients would choose to die in hospital, Thomas et al.[16] have recently illustrated how patients recognise that preferred place of death is contingent on many factors and is a fluid concept. Whilst improving services in the community and increasing access to hospice beds out of hours are clearly important aims, hospital admission will remain necessary and should not automatically be seen as a failure in care.

In delivering services out of hours, a compromise is inevitable between what is optimal – i.e. continuous availability of the patient's own primary care team, which maintains regular contact with the patient, communicating effectively, accessing specialist advice and properly resourced community services when necessary, and acting promptly in any emergency situation – and what is achievable – i.e. an effective but less personal service. It is likely that there will always be difficulties in achieving what is both acceptable to the patient and carer, and what it is feasible to provide. Since exacerbating symptoms out of hours creates stress for patients and carers, expectations differ and effective service delivery depends on communication that is particularly challenging in the out-of-hours or emergency situation. Services that effectively manage one incident may be less effective in another. The search for effective solutions should take into account the complexities of palliative care in the community and the constraints of operating within a context of limited resources. Whilst commissioners and local providers should be encouraged to aim for the best, it is also important to realistically define and accept what is 'good enough'.

### Acknowledgements

The Scottish study was conducted by the Primary Palliative Care Research Group, in the Division of Community Health Sciences, the University of Edinburgh. Scott Murray was the principal grantholder and Marilyn Kendall conducted the interviews.

The English study was conducted as part of a research degree thesis, supervised by Dr Frances Griffiths, Warwick Medical School.

---

### Summary

- Few studies have examined patients' perspectives in out-of-hours palliative care.

- Calls out of hours are often complex.

- The presenting issue is most commonly pain or other symptoms.

- Patients and carers may have difficulty in assessing relevance of symptoms and knowing when and who to call.

- Problems with access to care may result from complexities of service or patients not wanting to be 'a nuisance'.

- Patients value out-of-hours care from a professional who knows them.

- Patients may be reassured by knowing the service provider has specific information regarding their disease and treatment.

- Good communication with patients and carers helps to ensure a satisfactory outcome from the patient and carer perspective.

- Complexities arising from unpredictable illness trajectories, social context and service-related factors suggest that the perfect solution may be elusive.

---

**REFERENCES**

1. Department of Health. *Patient and Public Involvement in the New NHS*. London: HMSO, 1999.

2. Scottish Executive. *Patient Focus and Public Involvement*. Edinburgh: Scottish Executive, 2003.

3. Worth A, Boyd K, Kendall M, Heaney D, Macleod U, Cormie P, Hockley J and Murray S. Out of hours palliative care: A qualitative study of cancer patients, carers and professionals. *British Journal of General Practice* 2006; **56**: 6–13.

4. Munday D and Griffiths F. Issues surrounding emergency admission of palliative care patients to general hospital beds [poster]. 8th Congress of the European Association for Palliative Care. 2–5 April 2003, The Hague, Netherlands

5. Shipman C, Payne F, Dale J and Jessop L. Patient-perceived benefits of and barriers to using out-of-hours primary care centres. *Family Practice* 2001; **18**: 149–55.

6. Payne F, Shipman C and Dale J. Patients' experiences of receiving telephone advice from a GP co-op. *Family Practice* 2001; **18**: 156–60.

7. McKinley R K, Stevenson K, Adams S and Manku-Scott T K. Meeting patient expectations of care: The major determinants of satisfaction with out-of-hours primary medical care? *Family Practice* 2002; **19**: 333–8.

8. Thomas K. Out of hours palliative care – bridging the gap. *European Journal of Palliative Care* 2000; **7**: 22–5.

9. Ewing G, Rogers M, Barclay S, McCabe J, Martin A and Todd C. Recruiting patients into a primary care based study of palliative care: Why is it so difficult? *Palliative Medicine* 2004; **18**: 452–9.

10. Shipman C, Addington-Hall J, Barclay S, Briggs J, Cox I, Daniels L, *et al.* Providing palliative care in primary care: How satisfied are GPs and district nurses with current out of hours arrangements? *British Journal of General Practice* 2000; **50**: 477–8.

11. Munday D, Dale J and Barnett M. Out of hours palliative care in the UK: Perspectives from general practice and specialist services. *Journal of the Royal Society of Medicine* 2002; **95**: 28–30.

12. Ingleton C, Morgan J, Hughes P, Noble B, Evans A and Clark D. Carer satisfaction with end-of-life care in Powys, Wales: A cross sectional survey. *Health and Social Care in the Community* 2004; **12**: 43–52.

13. King N, Bell D and Thomas K. Family carers' experiences of out of hours community palliative care: A qualitative study. *International Journal of Palliative Nursing* 2004; **10**: 76–83.

14. Thomas K. *Out of Hours Palliative Care in the Community*. London: Macmillan Cancer Relief, 2001.

15. Macmillan Cancer Relief. *The Gold Standard Framework Project*. London: Macmillan Cancer Relief, 2001.

16. Thomas C, Morris S and Clark D. Place of death: Preferences among cancer patients and their carers. *Social Science and Medicine* 2004; **58**: 2431–44.

CHAPTER | 6

# Continuity in specialist palliative care

*Dan Munday and Cathy Shipman*

## Introduction

Specialist palliative care services have undergone rapid expansion over the last 30 years as the principles of hospice care have been increasingly provided within the hospital and community setting as part of 'mainstream' NHS provision. Whilst initial aims were relatively modest in introducing palliative care services into areas where there had been none before, in the last 10 years there has been an increasing emphasis on palliative care for all regardless of diagnosis (malignant and non-malignant), in whatever setting (e.g. hospital, home or nursing home), whenever it is needed – i.e. 24-hour availability.[1-3]

The Cancer Plan published by the Department of Health in 2000[4] introduced the concept of 'supportive care', which includes psychosocial and spiritual support, and complementary therapies. Although it is not synonymous with palliative care the boundaries between them are blurred. Unlike palliative care, which was previously defined as relevant to patients with incurable disease,[5] such a restriction is not appropriate for supportive care that may be needed by a patient at any time in their disease trajectory. Furthermore, it is now recognised that palliative care itself is relevant earlier in the disease process, as the National Institute for Clinical Excellence (NICE) *Guidance on Cancer Services: Improving supportive and palliative care for adults with cancer* (2004) makes explicit:

> Palliative Care is the active holistic care of patients with advanced, progressive illness. Management of pain and other symptoms and provision of psychological, social and spiritual support is paramount. The goal of palliative care is achievement of the best quality of life for patients and their families. *Many aspects of palliative care are also applicable earlier in the course of the illness in conjunction with other treatments* [emphasis added].[6]

Extension of the concept and scope of palliative care in this way clearly has wide implications for specialist palliative care as supportive and palliative care now would seem to include anything that is not aimed at diagnosis and treatment of the underlying disease. This clearly needs to be considered whilst discussing continuity of care in specialist palliative care, although we will largely concentrate on provision for patients with advanced, progressive and life-limiting illness.

Exploring continuity in the context of specialist palliative care within this chapter, we will consider the complexity of the issues involved. This will include an examination of what we consider to be the barriers to effective continuity of care. We will review what research evidence is available surrounding continuity within specialist palliative care and look at some models that have been described and evaluated. Finally we will review the NICE guidelines for palliative care.

At the outset, however, we will explore the concept of specialist palliative care in general and from this look at continuity of specialist palliative care in particular.

### Specialist palliative care in the UK

As specialist palliative care has developed in the UK, it has expanded from its original structure within hospices to include support and advisory teams working within the community and hospital setting. Palliative care services can now be categorised as follows:

- in-patient facilities
- day care facilities
- hospice home care services
- Community Specialist Palliative Care Support Teams
- Hospital Specialist Palliative Care Support Teams.

This is rather an oversimplified categorisation since there is a large degree of variation within these basic definitions and there is often a large amount of overlap between the different categories. For instance, in-patient facilities may vary from isolated hospice units to specialist palliative care wards attached to cancer centres within large teaching hospitals. They may have varying degrees of specialist medical input, from those led by GPs with special interest in palliative care to services with a full complement of consultants in palliative medicine. Community and hospital specialist palliative care teams may work in isolation, with clinical nurse specialists (CNS) providing a service with little or no support from consultants in palliative medicine whilst others are led by consultant medical staff. Some teams may function as outreach teams from hospices with integral management structures; others may have little contact with in-patient units. Such variation has been highlighted in the study led by Skilbeck, Clark and Seymour into the work of Macmillan nurses.[7-9] (Macmillan nurses are palliative care CNSs, supported by the UK charity Macmillan Cancer Support. The terms CNS in palliative care and Macmillan nurse are often used interchangeably.)

Whilst the core members of the multidisciplinary team in specialist palliative care may comprise physicians and CNSs, other professionals are also often part of the team, including social workers, counsellors, physiotherapists, occupational therapists, chaplains, psychologists, etc. The exact make-up of each team is highly variable. Lack of uniformity in the configuration of palliative care services has been described by Ahmed et al. as resulting from 'the rapid and unplanned growth of hospices and other palliative care services'.[10]

In addition to the lack of uniformity of professionals within teams there is also a lack of consistency in how teams operate. Seymour et al. discovered that in teams comprising Macmillan nurses and consultants in palliative medicine, there was a variation in how services were delivered, sometimes leading to tensions and problems in 'delineating role boundaries'. In some teams, however, where interdisciplinary working relationships had been 'established particularly clearly ... enhanced collaboration and smooth relationships seem to be the result'.[9] Palliative care teams will often aspire to operate in a non-hierarchical manner, with each professional group respecting the perspective and skills of the others.[11] However, Clark and Seymour point out that whilst in palliative care teamwork 'barriers between disciplines are said to be lowered or even dismantled completely ... the extent to which this has been achieved has not however been subjected to critical scrutiny' (p. 83).[12]

The National Council for Palliative Care (NCPC) has delineated the differences between 'specialist palliative care', which is defined

as the work of those for whom palliative care is their core speciality, and the 'palliative care approach', which should be taken by all
healthcare professionals caring for patients with end-stage disease
(see Box 6.1).[5] However, the exact nature of specialist palliative care
is difficult to define, unlike specialities such as surgery, oncology,
radiology, etc. where the specialist activity is highly technical and
specific.[13] Furthermore, specialist palliative care is not focused on
one particular system, as in cardiology, or task, such as in oncology,
where the aim is to effect cure or regression in the disease, but on a
stage in the patient's condition[14] and the somewhat nebulous remit
of 'management of pain and other symptoms and provision of psychological, social and spiritual support'. As the scope of specialist
palliative care extends into other areas such as non-cancer illnesses,
issues of definition and scope are further compounded necessitating
further exploration and debate.

---

Box 6.1 **Differences between specialist palliative care and the
palliative care approach**

*Specialist palliative care services* are those services with palliative care as their
core speciality. Specialist palliative care services are needed by a significant
minority of people whose deaths are anticipated. It may be provided either:

■ directly or

■ indirectly through advice to a patient's present professional advisers/carers.

*The palliative care approach* aims to promote both physical and psychological
wellbeing. It is a vital and integral part of all clinical practice, whatever the
illness or its stage, informed by a knowledge and practice of palliative care
principles.

---

*Source*: NCHSPC.[5]

## Contexts for specialist palliative care

When palliative care was focused on terminal care within an institution, as in the early hospices (post-1967), palliative care (or hospice
care as it was then known) took place within its own context. Since
palliative care has extended its remit to the community and hospital
settings, where the vast majority of cancer patients spend the bulk of
their last year of life, the speciality is operating within a wider con-

text and necessarily working alongside other specialist and generalist healthcare professionals. In these situations, specialist palliative care practitioners do not take primary responsibility for the patient. This will reside with the GP (or technically now the primary care team) for patients in the community and the responsible consultant and his or her team within a hospital setting.

Palliative care in the UK provides a supportive role outside of hospice institutions, with the primary caring role being taken by other practitioners. Combined with a degree of ambiguity about the exact role of specialist palliative care and the extension of palliative care to an earlier point within the patient's disease trajectory, there is a lack of clarity with regard to what specialist palliative care should take responsibility for providing in any given situation.[15] This is particularly problematic as individual practitioners and teams may have different understanding, perspectives and practices surrounding this issue.[16,17] Patient care may become very complex with many different healthcare providers being involved, leading to problems in communication and the possibility of care duplication in some aspects and failure in others (see Figure 6.1).

Figure 6.1 **Professional roles in palliative care**

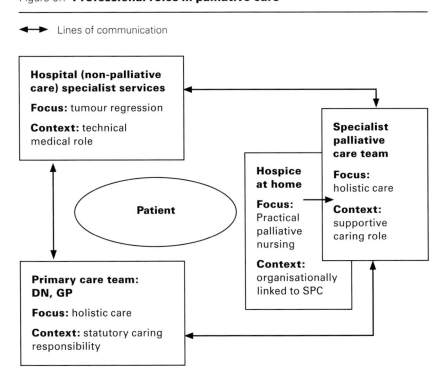

Such complexity may be less apparent in palliative care systems in some other countries, notably the USA[18] and also Australia.[19] In these contexts, when terminally ill patients are referred, the palliative care team takes on the primary caring role. Particularly in the USA with its relatively poorly developed primary care services, family doctors may be rarely involved in care of the terminally ill.[20] In addition, since rules for palliative care provision by Medicare in the USA require that patients forgo any curative treatment, there is no defined role for the oncologist.[21] Comparisons between services offered in these countries in terms of continuity of care need to be made with these contextual differences in mind.

**Continuity and specialist palliative care**

Whilst continuity of care is necessary to prevent the patient receiving treatment in a disjointed and inappropriate fashion, it is not a discrete property of patient care, but rather is an important element of all good care. Haggerty *et al.* point out that connected and coherent care is necessary for continuity to exist, but that 'continuity is how individual patients experience integration of services and co-ordination'.[22] The patient's experience of continuity, or lack of it, is also contingent on many factors, not only coordination and integration of services. Ultimately no objective measure of continuity at the level of the individual patient exists. Since continuity is such a fundamental aspect of care, it is perhaps most noticeable by its absence rather than its presence. (See Chapter 1 for a full exploration of this.)

Several studies have highlighted problems that occur when there is lack of continuity. Jarrett *et al.* reported a qualitative interview study of terminally ill patients and their lay carers, in which lack of continuity was an emergent theme. Large numbers of nursing professionals were involved with patients, which led to problems with continuity and communication. New nurses would have to familiarise themselves with the patient's history and frequent changes in nursing staff would make it difficult for the patient and carer to build relationships with the nurse. Failure of communication between specialist and generalist providers was also evident, e.g. the GP not being notified when a patient was discharged.[23] Bestall and colleagues, in a discussion of the findings of an interview study with patients and healthcare professionals, also comment on the effect of large numbers of carers being involved with the patient. This might lead to a patient declining an appropriate change in management if it might threaten their relationship with a health professional.[24]

## Out-of-hours specialist palliative care

Since the majority of the week lies outside of normal working hours, to provide continuity of specialist palliative care some degree of out-of-hours provision is necessary. Hospice and specialist palliative care units will provide a 24-hour nursing service for their in-patients and will have provision for medical cover, although smaller units may need to rely on the services of other medical staff (such as local GPs) rather than their own doctors. Lack of out-of-hours services in hospital or community settings might lead to difficulties for non-specialist healthcare professionals in delivering appropriate care to palliative care patients.

Kendall and Jeffrey surveyed staff in a cancer centre about their experiences and preferences for out-of-hours palliative care. The majority of those surveyed agreed that there was a need for access to specialist palliative care out of hours, particularly for symptom control advice, which could be largely delivered over the telephone. Most respondents felt confident in dealing with problems overnight until the following day, but found managing problems for a whole weekend unacceptable.[25]

Since there is lack of uniformity of specialist palliative care services nationally it is likely that this will be matched by marked variation in forms of out-of-hours provision. In 1999 a survey of all medical directors of in-patient specialist palliative care and hospice units within the UK was undertaken to ascertain availability of out-of-hours admission to specialist palliative care beds, specialist palliative care advice and the barriers to providing such a service.[26] Two-hundred and twenty-four units were surveyed, with replies being received from 182 (81 per cent).

This study confirmed that smaller hospices were less likely to provide out-of-hours medical cover, with hospices of fewer than 10 beds, 10–19 beds and more than 20 beds being covered by their own doctors in 34 per cent, 66 per cent and 72 per cent of cases respectively.

Overall, 9 per cent *did not* accept any admissions (4 per cent more than 20 beds; 8 per cent, 10–19 beds; 16 per cent, fewer than 10 beds). Forty per cent would only take patients who were known to the unit. If any admissions were accepted out of hours, the majority (71 per cent) were at the discretion of the first on call; however, 24 per cent would only admit a patient after the agreement of a consultant. Only one specialist palliative care unit gave 'open access' to GPs for any eligible patients, i.e. similar to the traditional practice of a GP referring for surgical or medical admission out of hours.

When these medical directors were asked whether open access to GPs for admission of appropriate patients out of hours would be possible, 73 per cent said that this would need either major changes or would be impossible to provide. When asked what would be the major problems associated with offering open access, 53 per cent cited lack of finance, 62 per cent lack of staff and 53 per cent lack of beds. Comments indicated concerns associated with offering open access, notably: inappropriate admission, including patients who should have been admitted to acute medical wards; beds being blocked by social admissions; the disruption caused to the running of the hospice; and loss of control over admissions (Box 6.2). The single specialist unit that did offer open access commented positively that it worked well and did not lead to inappropriate admissions.

---

Box 6.2 **Opinion of Specialist Palliative Care Unit (SPCU) medical directors regarding potential problems of offering open access to GPs for SPCU beds**

- Inappropriate admissions.
- Social admissions.
- Blocking of beds.
- Need to cancel booked admissions.
- Inadequate nursing levels.
- 'Acute patients' would be admitted rather than to hospital.
- Loss of control over admissions.
- Disruption to the unit at night.
- Against 'hospice philosophy'.

In a parallel survey of GP out-of-hours cooperatives (see Chapter 2), medical directors of the cooperatives indicated that the need for emergency admission of patients into palliative care beds was an important issue, although only infrequently needed. Seventy-one per cent indicated that access to palliative care beds out of hours would be useful; however, many understood that there were major resource issues and general lack of hospice beds would lessen the likelihood of beds being available out of hours.

Asked about out-of-hours advice, 89 per cent of hospice medical directors said that they had such a service for GPs and 49 per cent had written to GPs to inform them of this service, the rest relying on newsletter or informal contact. Satisfaction with the advice service had been formally audited by 29 per cent. Comments regarding publicity concerning the advice service suggested that some medical directors were worried that this might result in the service being over-run with requests for help.

On the part of the cooperative medical directors, the majority responded positively regarding the quality of out-of-hours telephone advice services when they were available, but claimed that the need to access telephone advice was relatively infrequent.[26] This perception is supported by the results from an audit of a well-publicised telephone advice service in Leicester, in which only 93 calls were received in the first year of operation.[27]

In general it may therefore be concluded that, whilst out-of-hours specialist palliative care support is necessary both for community and hospital contexts, the absolute level of need has been small. What is not known is how the rapid and continuing changes in primary care provision in the UK over the last two years will affect the need for out-of-hours specialist palliative care. Anecdotal evidence is emerging that in some areas these recent changes have been detrimental to caring for palliative care patients, with increased demands being placed on specialist services to 'fill the gaps'.

### Models promoting continuity of specialist palliative care

Achieving continuity is a key aim of most specialist palliative care services, even if this is not explicit. Although it is a central feature that runs through all examples of good palliative care, it might not be the primary aim of service providers and might not be reported on directly in evaluative studies. We present the results from three studies in the UK in which a service has been instigated that is at least partly aimed at achieving continuity in different aspects of patient care.

### Coordination of care

Addington-Hall *et al.* report on a randomised controlled trial (RCT) using a nurse coordinator for terminally ill cancer patients.[28,29] This experimental study was carried out in a South London borough in 1987–90 and was established in recognition of the fact that, whilst some terminally ill patients and their families receive prompt and adequate services, others do not. The intervention under investigation involved the employment of nurse coordinators to 'broker' for patients. Their responsibilities included assessing the patient's need for services from the NHS, local authority or voluntary agencies, and to facilitate the provision of these services for the patient. The coordinator was to stay in contact with the patient and carers, and to monitor changing needs whilst the patient and carers were encouraged to contact her for help and advice. Clinical advice and practical nursing were not provided by the coordinator, but by usual providers, i.e. district nurses, Macmillan nurses, hospice services, etc. Patients were allocated to the intervention or control group according to the practice with which they were registered. The evaluation was performed by independent interviewers who were not informed which group the patient was in. These interviewers collected details on symptom issues (physical and psychological), quality of life, services accessed and satisfaction with services from patients and their informal carers.

Although 554 patients entered the trial, only 203 were able to be interviewed at base line and on at least one follow-up occasion. This was largely because of deterioration in condition, as is not unusual for studies involving palliative care patients. There was little difference in outcomes between the intervention and control groups in terms of symptom control, access to community services and satisfaction with services received, either by the patient or his or her informal carers.[29] However, the intervention group had significantly fewer in-patient days and home nurse visits, although it is unclear what the mechanisms for this effect were. The trialists did calculate that this represented a cost saving of between 4 : 1 and 8 : 1.[28] Whether this exact model would be effective in other areas would depend on contextual issues that are not addressed by the papers linked to this study. However, the principle of a key professional to encourage continuity for the patient and carer is clearly an important issue for services to consider (see section 'Current guidelines for palliative care', p. 113).

### *24-hour home care respite service*

Specialist palliative home care services fall under two broad categories. First, there are specialist advisory and supportive services, which are provided mostly by clinical nurse specialists, often with the support of a consultant in palliative medicine. Second, there are hospice home care respite services.

Home care respite services offer 'hands on' nursing care for terminally ill patients, with nurses spending shifts working in the patient's home, normally liaising with district nurses and general practitioners. Nurses delivering this type of service are normally qualified or auxiliary nurses, rather than clinical nurse specialists, although the service may be managed by clinical nurse specialists or fall within the general rubric of hospice or specialist palliative care services. These management arrangements may therefore offer a fast track to specialist involvement. Such services may fall into the category of 'intermediate care' being neither truly specialist nor primary care. In common with other intermediate care services a major part of their focus may be in preventing admission to secondary care facilities.

With the variety of models of care and the varying degrees of overlap between these respite services and specialist palliative care services, a description of a typical service is impossible. Furthermore, the NCPC report of national palliative care services for 2003/4,[30] which gathers data regarding levels of activity in specialist palliative care, is unable to distinguish clearly between types of service. However, it does estimate that 79 per cent of visits in the community are by clinical nurse specialists and only 13 per cent by trained or untrained nursing staff, suggesting that specialist advice services are more common than home care respite services.

Hockley cites the reasons for a home care respite service being appropriate for individual palliative care patients as including:

- lack of the extended family to help and support
- since the main carer devotes time to the person who is dying, members especially children may be losing out on the attention of a parent
- the patient may need constant caring, repositioning in bed
- a prolonged dying period can often leave carers, especially if they are elderly, feeling emotionally drained
- many families are afraid of death and are comforted with the presence of a team member in their home.[31]

Much of the literature describing home care respite services relates to the USA. These studies are likely to be of marginal relevance to the UK because of the major differences in the arrangement of health-care delivery between these two countries. The most thoroughly researched service in the UK is that of the Cambridge Hospital at Home service for palliative care, which was evaluated using an RCT methodology and reported in a series of papers.[32-34]

The Cambridge Hospital at Home for palliative care is described as a service with the aim of improving terminal care, increasing care provision and increasing patient choice by providing a 'hands on' nursing service. The team is described as comprising six qualified nurses, all with an interest in, and most with experience of, palliative care nursing. Two nursing auxiliaries were also employed and a nurse coordinator, with agency nurses being employed as required.[32,33] The service was available for all patients irrespective of diagnosis for the last two weeks of life and was available for respite care for patients with cancer, HIV/AIDS and motor neurone disease. During the period of study, 88 per cent of patients admitted to hospital at home services had a cancer diagnosis, with no specific detail given regarding the diseases suffered by those patients with a non-cancer diagnosis. The standard care available in Cambridge is described as 'care in hospital and hospice or care at home with input from GP, district nursing, Marie Curie nursing, Macmillan nursing, evening district nursing, social services, private care and a flexible care nursing service'.[33]

The primary aim of the RCT for this service was to determine whether or not patients receiving the Hospital at Home service were more likely to die at home. Applying standard methodology for RCT, including intention-to-treat analysis, failed to show any statistical difference in place of death between patients randomised to receive the service and those randomised to standard care. Patients who actually received the service, rather than merely being allocated to it, were statistically more likely to die at home than those in the control group (78 per cent vs 58 per cent).[32] Whilst home deaths could not be strictly demonstrated to increase following referral to this service (using stringent RCT criteria), various other features were investigated as secondary outcomes. It was found that fewer GP visits were made in the penultimate week of life for those patients receiving the service. District nurses indicated that patients receiving the service had better night care, GPs gave patients lower ratings for anxiety and depression, and carers reported less pain and nausea. For other aspects of care and symptom control there were no statistical differences between both groups.[33]

In a later questionnaire study of local GP and district nursing views of the service, the majority of respondents thought that the service was important because of its provision of 24-hour care, support for patients and family, and enabling patients to remain at home. The majority also rated support for themselves from another professional with palliative care experience as important and that the organisation of care had been made easier by the hospital at home service. The main problem respondents reported was a relative lack of availability as compared with other services.[34]

The studies of the effectiveness of the Cambridge Hospital at Home service are interesting in several aspects. They represent an attempt to evaluate the effectiveness of a home care service using an RCT methodology, which the investigating team identify as the gold standard for service evaluation as specifically indicated by McQuay in relation to palliative care services.[35] Whilst RCTs hold this status, they are notoriously difficult to undertake in palliative care, with difficulties in recruitment and high attrition rates of subjects confounding results as well as ethical issues necessitating compromises in study design. In addition, as McQuay acknowledges, the success of interventions such as hospital at home services in comparison with medical therapies 'depends more on local conditions and, indeed, on local enthusiasms. What works in one set of circumstances may not be right for another.' Hence the results from such an RCT may not be generalisable or even transferable to other services. Therefore even if this study had shown that hospital at home was effective in enabling patients to remain at home, it would not necessarily have provided evidence even for similar services in similar areas. Since no health system remains static it might be argued that the effectiveness as demonstrated through the RCT might not have been valid at a future date within the area in which it was conducted.

A further difficulty with this study is the lack of observational and qualitative data, without which a clear understanding of the hospital at home service and the local context is difficult to achieve. Such data would have strengthened the insights relating to the overall assessment of the value of the service and would have been useful, even given the lack of RCT evidence for effectiveness. Future evaluations of palliative care services, such as the Cambridge Hospital at Home service, could be undertaken using a complex intervention evaluation framework,[36] as the research team suggest in a subsequent discussion paper.[37] Such a programme includes observational and qualitative studies in addition to an RCT as part of the evaluation design. Complex intervention trials are a major undertaking in terms of time and resources, however, and the problem of generalisability to other contexts still remains.

### Hospice rapid response service

Crises for terminally ill patients at home are not uncommon and even with meticulous advanced planning of services unforeseen problems can occur, for example: a sudden deterioration in the patient's condition; informal carers' inability to cope with patient care due to increasing needs of the patient; and illness or anxiety in the carer. Crises may be temporary or they may lead to higher levels of care need. Patients in a crisis may be admitted to hospital or a hospice if services are not available at short notice.

King *et al.* describe and evaluate a 24-hour rapid response service set up in Inverness.[38] This service was staffed by hospice ward nurses and was available within a radius of 25 miles of the hospice.

Patients could be referred from district nurses or GPs in the community, and also from the hospital Macmillan nurses, in order to enable patients to be discharged urgently. When a call was received, a 'bank' nurse would be called in to allow a nurse to go out to the patient's home. The service would be available for 48 hours, after which time a review was made, the service being discontinued when existing services were able to cope, the patient died or was admitted to hospital or hospice.

As part of the development of the service an evaluation programme was designed to assess its effectiveness and contribution to meeting patients' needs. This used descriptive and interview methodologies, and examined the first year of operation of the service. Interviews with 45 health professionals (GPs, district nurses, clinical nurse specialists and managers) were designed to assess structure and organisation of the service both at the outset and the end of the study period. Records were kept for each patient receiving the service, noting reasons for referral and the type of care given. Views of referrers and service providers were sought by questionnaire and focus group, and the views and experiences of informal carers were explored in post-bereavement interviews. In addition, the impact of the service on hospital and hospice admissions was made by reviewing data for the year before the service was set up and during the period of evaluation.

During the evaluation period of one year 17 patients received the service. The response time was less than four hours in 66 per cent of referrals and for all episodes it was judged as being appropriate. Fourteen patients finally died at home, with three dying in the hospice and no hospital deaths in the group receiving the service. Half of the home deaths occurred whilst the service was involved with their care, the other half following discharge. Interviews with informal carers after bereavement indicated high levels of satisfaction, although this only involved carers in eight of the 17 cases and therefore may be biased. Carers reported fear at the responsibility of looking after a dying person, appreciated being able to hand over care and felt positive about the professional attitude and competence of the rapid response nurses.

Attempts to evaluate the effect on crisis admissions revealed that numbers were too small for a valid comparison. Given the complex nature of the issues involved, it would not have been possible to have made any conclusion regarding a direct effect of the service on crisis admissions, which the investigators acknowledge.

Despite district nurses having reservations at the outset with regard to how the service would work and what effect it would have on their role, following the first year of operation the professionals referring patients to the service reported that it worked well. Although the rapid response nurses were initially concerned about their possible lack of preparedness for delivering the service, they expressed confidence in their role at the end of the first year. Their main concerns, however, were with issues over which they had little control, e.g. poor access to drugs out of hours, times when they could not have responded if the service had been required because of staffing shortages and concerns over personal safety in travelling in adverse conditions.

Whilst this study does not attempt to prove the effectiveness of the service through comparison with a control group, it does give a detailed picture of the service developed and assesses its impact in a variety of ways. These illustrate that the service was highly valued by both carers and community health professionals. It is also not unreasonable to believe that at least some of the patients given the service avoided a hospital admission. Clearly the effectiveness of any service such as this or any community respite service will be determined by local factors and it may be more appropriate to develop services in a rigorous manner, using a flexible approach to evaluation and using results to develop the service further.[39]

### Current guidelines for palliative care

In 2004 following two years of preparation including several draft editions circulated for consultation, the NICE *Guidance on Cancer Services: Improving supportive and palliative care for adults with cancer* was published. This document is based on research evidence and addresses clinical effectiveness and service delivery. Continuity of care is emphasised at the outset with the first chapter covering the need for coordinated care:

> People with cancer may require supportive and palliative care at different stages of the patient pathway and from a range of service

providers in the community, hospitals, hospices, care homes and community hospitals. This means that services need to work closely together to ensure that patients' and carers' needs are addressed with no loss of continuity (p. 35).[6]

The theme of continuity recurs throughout the document as a *leitmotif*. In particular it introduces the concept of the 'key worker' within the specialist palliative care team, defined as the 'person who, with the patient's consent and agreement, takes a key role in co-ordinating the patient's care and promoting continuity, ensuring the patient knows who to access for information and advice' (p. 204). The key worker may be a specialist nurse, social worker or allied health professional with the task of:

- orchestrating assessments to ensure patients' needs are elicited
- ensuring care plans have been agreed with patients
- ensuring findings from assessments and care plans are communicated to others involved in a patient's care
- ensuring patients know who to contact when help or advice is needed, whether the 'key worker' or other appropriate personnel
- managing transitions of care (p. 42).

The guidelines acknowledge, however, that evaluation of different models of key worker is desirable, since the role of a formal key worker is relatively poorly developed within specialist palliative care.

In addition specialist palliative care should be available throughout the week, including out of hours:

The team should be staffed to a level sufficient to undertake face-to-face assessments of all people with cancer at home or in hospital, 09.00 – 17.00, seven days a week. In addition, there should be access to telephone advice at all times (24 hours, seven days a week). This is considered a minimum level of service. Provision for bed-side consultations in exceptional cases outside the hours of 09.00 – 17.00, seven days a week is also desirable (p. 129).

The progress of specialist palliative care teams and Cancer Networks in implementing programmes to achieve continuity and 24-hour access to care, along with other aspects of specialist palliative care provision, are now monitored against standards developed from these guidelines.

## Conclusions

Provision of palliative care is complex, involving many services that need to be well coordinated and locally specific in order to meet the needs of patients. Continuity of specialist palliative care is an important aspect of delivering such a service and this is recognised by current guidelines for the delivery of palliative care. Problems that require specialist advice can occur at any time. This provides a challenge for specialist palliative care services, many of which are already stretched in the provision of a service in normal working hours. Commissioning of specialist palliative care services will need to be seen as a priority by Primary Care Trusts (PCT) if the aspirations for a comprehensive service are to be realised. In addition, integrated strategic planning across the primary and secondary care interface, between community and hospital services, and between the NHS and voluntary sector, is of paramount importance (see Chapter 10).

Occasionally patients who need specialist palliative care will need to be admitted out of hours. At present in many areas, hospices and specialist palliative care units are unable to offer admission to such patients and, even where such a service is available, a lack of available beds will often prevent such admissions. This inevitably leads to hospital admission for some patients, which may not always be the most appropriate context for their management.

Another approach to the lack of specialist in-patient beds would be to enable some patients to remain at home by developing enhanced home care nursing services, so that an appropriate level of professional nursing care is not only available for in-patients. Several different models have been suggested and evaluated in a variety of ways. Services need to be developed that link in with other locally available services, avoiding duplication of provision on the one hand and lack of specific service on the other. Current policies for avoiding hospital admission and affording patients the opportunity to remain at home, if that is their wish,[40] should encourage the development of community specialist palliative care services if such services are judged as effective in achieving these aims.

Given the local complexities involved in configuring and delivering community palliative care services, it is unlikely that their effectiveness can be usefully demonstrated using experimental methods such as the RCT. However, it is perhaps reasonable to ask along with Keeley:

> If we want to know whether five years of pill taking for high blood pressure will reduce our risk of stroke we are unwise to rely on our own or our doctor's common sense impression and want evidence from randomised controlled trials. But if our loved one is dying and wishes to die at home, how much evidence do we need that skilled home nursing available round the clock would be a good idea?[41]

If we can make the reasonable assumption that home care nursing and access to out-of-hours specialist advice is appropriate and desirable, the development and evaluation of palliative care services on a local level using a range of quantitative and qualitative methods should be encouraged. Using this model, the most appropriate local service may then be provided within the constraints of available resources and examples of good practice can be shared.

### Acknowledgement

We would like to thank Dr Sally Johnson for her helpful comments during the preparation of this chapter.

---

### Summary

- Continuity in specialist palliative care is a complex issue.

- Specialist services need to work effectively with primary and relevant secondary services to provide continuity.

- Specialist services vary greatly between localities for historical and contextual reasons.

- No single model for effective continuity in specialist palliative care exists.

- Effective services providing continuity need to be locally developed and evaluated.

- Continuity is a central feature identified in the National Institute for Health and Clinical Excellence (NICE) guidelines for palliative care.

---

### REFERENCES

1. *Dilemmas and Directions: The future of specialist palliative care.* London: National Council for Hospice and Specialist Palliative Care, 1997.

2. DoH. *EL(96)85 A Policy Framework for Commissioning Cancer Services: Palliative care services.* London: NHS Executive, 1996.

3. Tebbit P. *Palliative Care 2000: Commissioning through partnership.* London: National Council for Hospices and Specialist Palliative Care, 1999.

4. DoH. *The NHS Cancer Plan: A plan for investment, a plan for reform.* London: Department of Health, 2000.

5. NCHSPC. *Specialist Palliative Care: A statement of definitions.* London: National Council for Hospice and Specialist Palliative Care Services, 1995 (Occasional Paper vol. 8).

6. NICE. *Guidance on Cancer Services: Improving supportive and palliative care for adults with cancer.* London: National Institute for Clinical Excellence, 2004.

7. Skilbeck J, Corner J, Bath P, *et al.* Clinical nurse specialists in palliative care. Part 1. A description of the Macmillan nurse caseload. *Palliative Medicine* 2002; **16**: 285–96.

8. Clark D, Seymour J, Douglas H-R, *et al.* Clinical nurse specialists in palliative care. Part 2. Explaining diversity in the organization and costs of Macmillan nursing services. *Palliative Medicine* 2002; **16**: 375–85.

9. Seymour J, Clark D, Hughes P, *et al.* Clinical nurse specialists in palliative care. Part 3. Issues for the Macmillan nurse role. *Palliative Medicine* 2002; **16**: 386–94.

10. Ahmed N, Bestall J, Ahmedzai S, Payne S, Clark D and Noble B. Systematic review of the problems and issues of accessing specialist palliative care by patients, carers and health and social care professionals. *Palliative Medicine* 2004; **18**: 525–42.

11. Hoy A. Teamworking in Palliative Care. *European Journal of Palliative Care* 2005; **12**: 227.

12. Clark D and Seymour J. *Reflections on Palliative Care: Sociological and policy perspectives.* Buckingham: Open University Press, 1999.

13. Robbins M. Assessing needs and effectiveness: Is palliative care a special case? In: Clark D, Hockley J and Ahmedzai. S, eds. *New Themes in Palliative Care*. Buckingham: Open University Press, 1997.

14. Doyle D. Palliative medicine – a time for definition. *Palliative Medicine* 1993; **3**: 253–5.

15. Clark D. Between hope and acceptance: The medicalisation of dying. *British Medical Journal* 2002; **324 (7342)**: 905–7.

16. Field D. Special not different: General practitioners' accounts of their care of dying people. *Social Science and Medicine* 1998; **46 (9)**: 1111–20.

17. Shipman C, Addington-Hall J, Barclay S, *et al.* How and why do GPs use specialist palliative care services? *Palliative Medicine* 2002; **16 (3)**: 241–6.

18. Hearn J and Higginson I. Do specialist palliative care teams improve outcomes for cancer patients? A systematic literature review. *Palliative Medicine* 1998; **12**: 317–32.

19. Mitchell G, Reymond E and McGrath B. Palliative care: Promoting general practice participation. *Medical Journal of Australia* 2004; **180**: 207–8.

20. Gwinn R. Family physicians should be experts in palliative care. *American Family Physician* 2000; **61 (3)**: 641–2.

21. Medicare Hospice Benefits [web page]. Available at: www.hospicenet. org/html/medicare.html [accessed March 2007].

22. Haggerty J, Reid R, Freeman G, Starfield B, Adair C and McKendry R. Continuity of care: A multidisciplinary review. *British Medical Journal* 2003; **327**: 1219–21.

23. Jarrett N, Payne S and Wiles R. Terminally ill patients' and lay carers' perceptions and experiences of community based service. *Journal of Advanced Nursing* 1999; **29**: 476–83.

24. Bestall J, Ahmed N, Ahmedzai S, Payne S, Noble B and Clark D. Access and referral to specialist palliative care: Patients' and professionals' experiences. *International Journal of Palliative Nursing* 2004; **10**: 381–9.

25. Kendall C and Jeffrey D. Out-of-hours specialist palliative care provision in an oncology centre: Is it worthwhile? *Palliative Medicine* 2003; **17**: 461–4.

26. Munday D, Dale J and Barnett M. Out of hours palliative care in the UK: Perspectives from general practice and specialist services. *Journal of the Royal Society of Medicine* 2002; **95**: 28–30.

27. Lloyd-Williams M and Rashid A. An analysis of calls to an out-of-hours palliative care advice line. *Public Health* 2003; **117**: 125–7.

28. Raftery J, Addington-Hall J M, MacDonald L, *et al.* A randomised controlled trial of the cost effectiveness of a district coordinating service for terminally ill cancer patients. *Palliative Medicine* 1996; **10**: 151–61.

29. Addington-Hall J M, MacDonald L, Anderson H, *et al.* Randomised controlled trial of effects of co-ordinating care for terminally ill cancer patients. *British Medical Journal* 1992; **305**: 1317–22.

30. NCPC. *National Survey of Patient Activity Data for Specialist Palliative Care Services: MDS full report for the year 2003–2004.* London: The National Council for Palliative Care, 2005.

31. Hockley J. The evolution of the hospice approach. In: Clark D, Hockley J, Ahmedzai S, eds. *New Themes in Palliative Care.* Buckingham: Open University Press, 1997.

32. Grande G E, Todd C J, Barclay S I G and Farquhar M C. Does hospital at home for palliative care facilitate death at home? Randomised controlled trial. *British Medical Journal* 1999; **319 (7223)**: 1472–5.

33. Grande G, Todd C, Barclay S and Farquhar M. A randomized controlled trial of a hospital at home service for the terminally ill. *Palliative Medicine* 2000; **14**: 375–85.

34. Todd C, Grande G, Barclay S and Farquhar M. General practitioners' and district nurses' views of hospital at home for palliative care. *Palliative Medicine* 2002; **16**: 251–4.

35. McQuay H and Moore A. Need for rigorous assessment of palliative care. *British Medical Journal* 1994; **309**: 1315–16.

36. Campbell M, Fitzpatrick R, Haines A, *et al.* Framework for Design and Evaluation of Complex Interventions to Improve Health. *British Medical Journal* 2000; **321**: 391–6.

37. Grande G and Todd C. Why are trials in palliative care so difficult? *Palliative Medicine* 2000; **14**: 69–74.

38. King G, Mackenzie J, Smith H and Clark D. Dying at home: Evaluation of a hospice rapid response service. *International Journal of Palliative Nursing* 2000; **6 (6)**: 280–7.

39. Ingleton C, Field D and Clark D. Formative evaluation and its relevance to palliative care. *Palliative Medicine* 1998; **12**: 197–203.

40. DoH. *Building on the Best: Choice, responsiveness and equity in the NHS.* London: Department of Health, 2003.

41. Keeley D. Rigorous assessment of palliative care revisited. *British Medical Journal* 1999; **319 (7223)**: 1447–8.

# CHAPTER 7

# Continuity of palliative care and the elderly

*Peter Ferry*

## Introduction

The WHO has recently highlighted the importance of improving access to palliative care for older people.[1] Referral to specialist palliative care services tends to be less frequent than for younger age groups. As an ageing population tends to suffer co-morbidities, and palliative care is more frequently conceptualised as appropriate for cancer sufferers, it is possible that the elderly experience inequitable access to generalist as well as specialist palliative care. Good coordination of services is important across primary, secondary, specialist and other health and social care sectors.[1]

Continuity of care is a multidimensional term used to describe a variety of relationships or outcomes between patients and the delivery of health care.[2,3] The care that people need over an extended period of time to address their physical and mental health needs as a result of disability, accident or illness is called 'continuing care' or 'long-term care'. This type of care may require transition from one level of service provided from the National Health Service (NHS) and/or Social Services (SS) to another.[4] Care can be provided in a wide range of settings and this is described below. Greater continuity of care reduces hospitalisations,[5,6] improves follow-up, increases patient and staff satisfaction, promotes compliance with recommended care, reduces duplication of tests, and reduces readmission rates to hospital.[2,7-13]

The National Service Framework (NSF) for Older People[14] has therefore emphasised that care needs of older people should be given priority. It has identified potential ways of improving continuity of care. Intermediate care developments, such as rapid response teams and supported discharge from hospital, require collaboration between organisations. NHS and social service joint working is a key aspect of the programme and the Single Assessment Process (SAP) requires joint cooperation between agencies. This chapter will look at how well the NSF supports care of older people and, in particular, to what extent it provides for their palliative care needs. It will present models of good practice in providing continuity of palliative care to older people. It will look at nursing and residential care, and support at home. It will also identify gaps in provision including adequate resource allocation for care at the end of life.

## Background

Over the past 20 years there has been a dramatic increase in the population of older people in relation to the world population growth. This change has occurred more markedly in the very old (>80 year olds) where there has been a 69 per cent increase compared with an increase in the total world population of 38 per cent. Social, economic and political implications result from such a disproportionate growth. The consequences to the individual older patient are the complexities of multiple pathology and the subsequent care needs that usually follow.

The complex nature of problems faced by most older people warrants a multidisciplinary approach. What may start as a physical problem can very quickly result in a social, psychological or spiritual problem or a combination of these. Older people tend to be heavy users of the most costly health services, including hospitalisation, nursing home and social care.[2,15,16] With policies aimed at reducing hospital stays, there can, unfortunately, be less time for older people to rehabilitate adequately and to return to their previous level of functioning.[17-20] Of greater concern can be where there is little time to prepare an individual for an impending institutional placement decision or even involvement in the decision making.[13]

In the UK it is estimated that patients with advanced cancer (most of whom are elderly) spend approximately 90 per cent of their time under the care of the GP at home rather than in hospitals or institutions. Most people with a terminal illness would prefer to die at home but most people are dying in hospital or institutions and only a third of patients are dying at home.[21-6] An article by Gott et al.[27] has redefined the concept of 'home' in this context to mean more than a physical location, but an area representing familiarity, comfort and the presence of loved ones. While many elderly people die in hospitals, a greater proportion die in nursing and care homes than do younger palliative care patients.[28] Some research suggests that in the elderly fear of dying alone or being a burden on family members might incline a preference towards dying in a hospice or even hospital.[29] Practical problems in caring for the elderly dying at home include absence of informal carers, and problems associated with intimate care being given by the patient's children.

When considering the palliative care needs of older people one needs to be aware of the multiple chronic degenerative diseases that occur in addition to their terminal illness. Examples of such co-morbidities are degenerative diseases (such as osteoarthritis), neurological diseases (such as stroke or Parkinson's disease – although these can have terminal phases) and depression. Failure to recognise and manage these co-morbid conditions will result in unnecessary suffering. Older people commonly present to the healthcare professional with the so called 'geriatric giants': immobility, instability, incontinence or intellectual deterioration. One needs to take note that these are symptom complexes rather than diagnoses. Every effort should be made to arrive at a cause or list of causes for the problem in question, rather than attributing all these symptom complexes to old chronological age.

In a typical frail older patient with a terminal illness such as cancer, one will usually encounter more than one of these 'geriatric giants'. It must be emphasised that the cumulative burden of these pathologies results in a multiplier effect on the patient's disability. In addition, since taking more than three different drugs is common in this age group the probability of adverse drug interactions is high.

The main terminal diagnoses for older people are cancer (half of all cancer in the West is present in people > 65 years of age),[30] congestive cardiac failure (the leading cause of death in the UK), chronic renal failure, respiratory failure and cerebrovascular failure including delirium and dementia. Multiple co-morbidities can make it difficult to identify a primary cause of death. In addition, with palliative care often being linked to specific diagnoses, through specialist services focusing on cancer and NSFs being disease specific, elderly patients with complex co-morbidities might not be identified as needing palliative care.

It is very important to manage patients with terminal non-cancer diagnoses with the same level of palliative care expertise as cancer patients. A central difficulty, however, is to determine when a non-cancer diagnosis is a palliative or terminal one. This is partly because with advanced treatment regimes people are now living longer with such diseases, but also because non-cancer disease trajectories often follow a regular 'relapse–remission' course (as in respiratory or heart disease) or a gradual decline as in dementia (see Figure 7.1). Physical palliation in heart and respiratory disease is also quite different from that in cancer, as it is principally through disease modification. These issues can make it difficult for the health professional to accept that all these diagnoses should receive the same palliative care approach or to be aware of when it becomes most appropriate to adopt such an approach. Research has shown considerable need for symptom control and psychosocial support in patients suffering from non-malignant conditions, most of whom are elderly, as well as needs for family support, greater communication and choice concerning end of life care.[31-3]

**Current position**

The Community Care Act (1990) was intended to stimulate the development of flexible services to enable people to remain properly supported in their own homes.[34] Following its implementation there were reports of shifting boundaries between health and social services, and inequitable assessment of need and financial responsibility for care in different parts of the UK.[26,35]

The recent revision of the Continuing Care NHS health policy is an opportunity to ensure that people get access to the health and social care they need, in a timely fashion with the NHS paying for the health components of the care package. Primary Care Trusts (PCTs) are expected to arrange, fund and meet the continuing health needs of their population, from primary health care to specialist healthcare support, rehabilitation, community health services, respite health care and palliative care among others. Individual Strategic Health Authorities define their own eligibility criteria according to categories set out in the Continuing Care (NHS Responsibilities) Directions 2003 (Box 7.1).[36]

Figure 7.1 **Typical illness trajectories for people with progressive chronic illness**

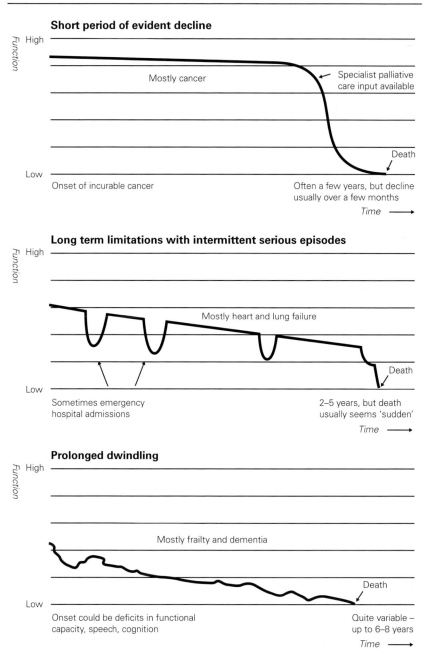

**Short period of evident decline**

Function — High

Mostly cancer

← Specialist palliative care input available

Death

Low

Onset of incurable cancer

Often a few years, but decline usually over a few months

Time ⟶

**Long term limitations with intermittent serious episodes**

Function — High

Mostly heart and lung failure

Death

Low

Sometimes emergency hospital admissions

2–5 years, but death usually seems 'sudden'

Time ⟶

**Prolonged dwindling**

Function — High

Mostly frailty and dementia

Death

Low

Onset could be deficits in functional capacity, speech, cognition

Quite variable – up to 6–8 years

Time ⟶

*Source*: Murray S A, Kendall M, Boyd K and Sheikh A. Illness trajectories and palliative care. *British Medical Journal* 2005; **330**: 1007–11. Adapted from Lynn and Adamson.

---

Box 7.1 **West Midlands South Strategic Health Authority eligibility criteria for continuing health and social care**[37]

The test for eligibility for continuing NHS healthcare will be met when:

**1** The complexity or intensity of their medical, nursing or other clinical care needs (and any combination of these needs) or the need for frequent, not easily predictable, interventions requires the supervision of a consultant, or other NHS clinician.

**2** Where an individual has a rapidly deteriorating or unstable medical, physical or mental condition.

**3** Where an individual is in the final stages of a terminal illness and likely to die in the near future.

**4** Where an individual's health needs require the routine use of specialist healthcare equipment under the supervision of NHS staff.

**5** Where the individual requires non-registered nursing care to the extent that goes beyond what can properly be described as incidental or ancillary to the accommodation and personal care needs.

---

In practice, however, the complexities of individual patients' situations are such that they do not fit easily into well-defined criteria. For example, in the advanced stages of heart failure, patients are usually ill for many months or years with occasional acute, severe exacerbations, each of which can result in death. It is very difficult to predict such a patient's illness trajectory over six weeks in comparison with a patient suffering from cancer, who typically follows a reasonably predictable decline.

## Striving for good practice

### Quality of care

Continuity of care is a critical component of quality patient care for all patient groups including older people. The extent to which a good standard of continuity of care is being achieved is difficult to quantify as there is a paucity of reliable and valid instruments to measure the quality of continuing care.[38] It has been suggested that the focus of quality in continuity of care should be on patient outcomes regardless of structure and process.[30] Thus patients' perspectives should be the driving force for monitoring quality in this field. Others take this a step further and argue that not only the patients' physical, psychosocial and spiritual wellbeing should be considered, but also the patients' family wellbeing and their perceptions of care.[39] One author[40] states that services for dying patients are an indicator of the overall quality and compassion of those who provide them. While not all may agree, many consider that high-quality palliative care in any environment can virtually eliminate requests for voluntary euthanasia.[41]

Recent national standards and frameworks for good practice promoting continuity within palliative care have been established (Box 7.2). Further research is needed to assess their relevance and develop their potential for an elderly population suffering from multiple co-morbidities.

---

**Box 7.2 Standards and frameworks promoting continuity in palliative care (see Chapter 11)**

**1** *National Institute for Health and Clinical Excellence* (NICE) guidelines on supportive and palliative care provides an evidence-based assessment on which to develop palliative care services.[42]

**2** *Macmillan Gold Standards Framework* (GSF) aims to improve palliative care provided by the primary care team. It enables terminally ill patients to be identified, their care needs assessed, and a plan of care with all the relevant agencies organised.[43]

**3** *Preferred Place of Care* (PPC) is a tool that enables healthcare professionals to discuss with patients and carers their preferences around end-of-life care to enable them to make informed choices.[44]

**4** *The Liverpool Care Pathway for the Dying* (Marie Curie Cancer Care) is a tool that assists healthcare professionals to deliver high-quality care as the end of life approaches. It is used both in cancer and in older people dying from a range of other conditions.[45]

---

### Support for patients and relatives

Changing family structures mean that more older people now live alone and apart from their immediate and extended family. Caring for an ill patient at home requires considerable and continuous energy, effort and time on the part of carers. Most informal carers tend to be older women, who might be frail themselves and physically and emotionally exhausted. One can support carers by offering respite care, providing sufficient resources and support, and preventative education to limit the impact of the caring role.[21] Support for both patients and carers should ideally be given in any setting that both parties feel most comfortable with. Some patients worry about their family carers becoming distressed at witnessing their own suffering, while others do not like being a burden to their family. The place where a patient is cared for is perhaps less important than the patient's and family's experience of the caring process itself.[46]

Caring for patients' relatives should extend to the time after death, particularly in home care when the family had been the main carers, and bereavement support should also be a component part of any package of care.[47] Providing sufficient support to carers can lead to a greater chance of continuity of care at home as research has shown that, when care becomes a burden, the patient is more likely to be admitted to an institution.[48] Continuity of care concerns both informal and formal care, and often requires a complex network of support.

Older people who have to be relocated due to their continuing care needs can suffer from the 'relocation stress syndrome', which is a set of physiological and psychosocial disturbances that result from the transfer from one environment to another. Thus older people who are being relocated should be supported fully all the way from pre-discharge to post-discharge.[13]

### Planning

When the older patient is terminally ill, planning should take on a different dimension with meticulous attention to detail. A small number of patients who are terminally ill make several transitions between different care settings or service providers. Negative impacts of such multiple transitions may result in discontinuity of care, poor coordination of care, possible financial burden and psychological distress.[49] One must strive to avoid crises that require trips to the emergency department or long stays in hospital.[50]

Good hospital discharge planning is vital for this vulnerable population. The most vulnerable groups are those who live alone, those who rely on many community services and those with multiple co-morbidities independent of age.[51] A study has shown high levels of satisfaction in involving older people and their carers in discharge planning.[52] Various strategies for discharge planning can be used to promote continuity of care between hospital and community services,[52,53] as discussed below.

There has been a concern with older patients remaining in acute hospital beds (labelled somewhat inappropriately bed blocking) over recent years and suggestions proposed as to how this problem can be solved. Some authors argue that there is a lack of expertise in general wards to assess disability, expedite negotiated discharges or reliably identify continuing care needs in older people with complex problems, and that a multidisciplinary approach with input from a consultant in elderly care important.[35] However, the main reasons for considerable delay in discharging older people from hospital usually originate from administrative or organisational issues that are compounded by social services resource constraints.[54] On the other hand, however, there is little evidence to show that patients who are inappropriately 'blocking hospital beds' would have had better outcomes if they had been discharged earlier as these patients may indeed be appreciably very unwell.[55] An increasingly ageing population in coming years is likely to further compound these problems.[56]

## Problematic areas

### Continuity of care in non-cancer diagnoses

Older people require palliative care not just for a cancer diagnosis, but also more commonly for a major organ failure such as heart failure and neurodegenerative diseases (such as dementia, stroke, Parkinson's disease). Such patients have an illness trajectory that is not as linear as a cancer.[33,57,58] leading to unpredictability that can make long-term care planning very difficult for such patients. Three typical illness trajectories have been described for patients with progressive chronic illness: that of cancer, organ failure and the trajectory for the frail elderly or those with dementia (see Figure 7.1).[58]

Prognostic optimism by healthcare professionals is not uncommon. This tends to prolong the use of potentially curative therapy despite the production of symptoms contributing to an adverse quality of life.[59] This is potentially problematic for patients as palliative care services may not be available to them or, if they are available, in some instances are poorly coordinated.[60]

### Difficulties in access to care

A multidisciplinary assessment will help to identify the person's and family's physical, social, emotional and spiritual needs. A practical care plan based on the patient's needs and informed by the likely trajectory that the patient's illness will follow should be made.
Holistic care should include:

1. Clinical care, including access to primary and specialist services, domiciliary services, nursing care, access to in-patient care for respite care or for symptom control, equipment to provide symptom control

2. Supportive care, which includes home care, long-term residential care, equipment for the home, e.g. adjustable height beds, hoist, etc.

There have been reports of inadequate provision for the elderly in care homes with lack of quality and appropriateness.[20,35,61] This may be due to the reduction in the number of care homes[20,62] and staff shortages for both residential and care home services.

### Lack of continuity of care

Continuity of care for the elderly has been cited as poor in all health-care settings.[40, 63-5] Similar problems exist in other countries where fragmentation of care seems to be the main problem.[66-8] One interesting solution for this problem has been described in which a user-led daily living plan was developed by older people in partnership with health and social care professionals. This person-centred model facilitated interagency communication leading to high levels of satisfaction.[69]

## Moving forward

### *What are we aiming for?*

The goal of palliative care is to achieve the best possible quality of life for patients and their families.[70] From the users' perspective, patients would wish to be cared for in a dignified way,[25,71] having their loved ones nearby and having expert assistance when needed[23,72] in any environment that they are cared for.[73] From the families' perspective, informal carers need to be supported,[23,25] by adequate provision of respite care for the patient, enjoy good communication with health-care professionals[22,51] and have access to a good bereavement service after their loved ones have passed away.[23,74]

### Steps needed to move forward

The most important steps needed to move forward in providing continuity of care for older people in palliative care are coordination of care, adequate communication and cooperation between different providers of care so that the receivers enjoy seamless care.[16,18,25,35,67,75]

One of the problems in implementation can be territoriality between professions,[69] although difficulties can lie within the social structures of the respective organisations rather than with the individual professional. Continuity of care depends on the palliative care network to create effective teams at an interagency and interdisciplinary level.[76,77] Absence of this continuity across boundaries may not only result in increased morbidity but also possibly lead to increased mortality in vulnerable older people.[78]

The NSF for Older People[14] has made a commitment to introduce a Single Assessment Process (SAP)[79] for the comprehensive assessment of the health and social needs of older people and for better planning their care. The SAP is developed locally but is based on general principles, namely person-centred and interprofessional collaboration, taking account of external and environmental factors. Consent is obtained from the older person to share information between different agencies. The eventual plan is for the SAP to be in electronic format and shared between primary and secondary care and social services. Similar initiatives are available abroad.[80,81]

Discharge planning for older people needs to improve to promote continuity of care between hospital and community services. Various strategies can be applied such as the appointment of discharge coordinators in hospitals, hospital/community liaison nurses and the use of comprehensive assessment tools.[52, 82]

The multidisciplinary team approach in dealing with the complex issue of 'total suffering' (caused by a combination of physical, psychological, social, cultural and spiritual concerns) is the most logical one to follow.[30, 74] Teams should have a common goal, diversity of skills and knowledge, mutual support for team members and effective conflict management.[83] There is some evidence that comprehensive patient management by a multidisciplinary team improves the outcome for older patients hospitalised with congestive cardiac failure and patients with fractured neck of femur.[9, 87]

There are suggestions from the United States and Canada that a team 'case or care manager' coordinating multidisciplinary team involvement may act as an advocate and liaison officer for the patient and the family.[84, 85] Key workers may provide the best mechanism for information transfer and continuity of care across organisations (e.g. NHS and social services), across professions and across geographical boundaries.[86] Partnership between the multidisciplinary team, the patient and the patient's family in discharge planning has been shown to be very successful in providing good-quality continuity of care for older people.[87-90]

## Recommendations

### Person-centred care

At the heart of the NSF for Older People is the standard 'person-centred care'. However, the care for older people with advanced progressive illnesses is currently prioritised by diagnosis rather than need[57] and this goes against this principle. Access to palliative care continuing care services should be based on need not diagnosis,[90, 91] although there might be resource implications for those with longer-term frail trajectories.

### Education of healthcare professionals

All practitioners dealing with dying patients should be skilled in the 'palliative care approach'. However, teaching of palliative care is generally poor in medical schools and for junior medical staff in hospitals.[92] More education and training of healthcare professionals especially in communication skills is required so that they are able to discuss diagnosis, prognosis, treatment options and end-of-life care with their patients and their families.[21,87,93] Interdisciplinary training of healthcare professionals improves the understanding of the work environment 'on the other side' and helps to ensure a smooth transition on transferring patients across boundaries.[88,93,94]

### Improvement in human resources

The demographic trend of rising numbers of elderly people, and the nature of the trend in degenerative diseases that complicates terminal disease, is having an impact on the intensity of care required in older people who require continuing care. There is an urgent need to address the supply and efficient use of nursing staff skills in care homes.[95-7]

### Intermediate care

Intermediate care is an umbrella term that incorporates any service for older people that promotes a person's independence by providing enhanced services from the NHS and other local services to prevent unnecessary hospital admission,[98] enable early discharge from hospital and prevent premature or unnecessary admission to long-term residential care.[13] Similar initiatives are practised abroad.[98] There are various examples of how intermediate care can be run, for example social services residential rehabilitation schemes, support at home with intensive or rehabilitative home care, rapid-response team care at the patient's usual residence or residential/nursing home.[63] Intermediate care schemes were shown to be advantageous in lowering length of hospital stay, re-hospitalisation rates and improving patient satisfaction rates.[99] In practice, intermediate care schemes are working very efficiently and effectively in some areas, but not in others.

### Case/care management

Although a case management or key worker approach has the advantages of integration across disciplines, primary and secondary care, and health and social services provision of care[100] it may not be cost effective.[101] In the UK, this role may be undertaken by providers of intermediate care but leadership may be the missing link.[102] A further development on the managed care idea is the Kaiser Permanente model of telephone care coordination programme.[103] This was designed as a hospital-based, telephone-based programme run by qualified nursing staff for community-dwelling, chronically ill older people (over 65 years) who were either functionally impaired or socially isolated. The advantage with this system is that nurses could carry a much heavier caseload than other programmes that included clinic or home visiting. The disadvantages of such a system is that it potentially excludes people who are either deaf or cognitively impaired. In the UK, with a well-developed primary care system in comparison with that in the USA, such a monitoring system could be provided by adequately resourced community nursing services. However, major changes in the structure and delivery of primary care services within the UK are likely to be made in the near future and the exact role of the generic community nurse is at present uncertain.

### Patient record sharing

There is the potential of further developing the SAP into a shared electronic record (between all service providers) or a patient-held record.[104] A feedback loop system of communication across care settings, for example primary and secondary care, was proposed in one study.[76] The way this would work would be to investigate what types of information are required by each setting and whether or not the information is being transmitted and received. Standardised or collaborative care plans suitable and acceptable to both areas could then be established.

### Interagency collaboration

Integration and collaboration between key service providers such as health, social services and housing is seen by some to be the most important move in improving the continuum of care for older people.[105] Such a move has been initiated in the UK by the establishment of the Health and Social Care Joint Unit since the 1999 Health Act partnership. However, importantly, housing has not yet been integrated in the above collaboration. Housing managers have a huge stake in the decisions made by the NHS and social services as most decisions about continuing care for older people with palliative needs have a housing consequence.[106]

## Conclusion

Elderly patients have complex physical and psychosocial needs. Much ill health in the elderly population is related to several simultaneous disease processes plus a gradual decline in functioning related to the ageing process. In addition changes in the social structure mean that, increasingly, old people live alone with family who either live at a distance or are in full-time employment and unable to provide continuous care.

With high levels of non-malignant illness elderly people often receive inadequate palliative care, through lack of available services and disease trajectories with no clear terminal stage. The isolated elderly patient with poorly addressed health needs, inadequate and poorly coordinated social and supportive services is still a common feature of 21st century Britain.

The role of palliative care for the elderly is not clearly defined. There is a huge degree of overlap between what might be expected to be provided by generic medical and nursing services, specialist geriatric services and specialist palliative care services for the elderly. It could be argued therefore that for the frail elderly, whatever their diagnosis, even if it is due to frailty rather than a definable pathological process, a broadly palliative care approach should be taken. Certainly all care should be patient centred, holistic and integrated with attention to detail and good communication with patients and families, and between all healthcare providers. Whether this then can be classified specifically as palliative care or should be the mark of all good health care is open to question.

A common myth related to population ageing is that healthcare costs for older people will be overwhelming and unsustainable. This, however, assumes a consistent relationship between comparisons of the proportion a country spends on health care for older people and the proportion of older people in that country, which has not been shown internationally.[1] There is still time to plan for population ageing in terms of continuing care. Such new methods of continuing care should be person centred rather than service centred[107-9] and continuity of care should be multidimensional with interpersonal, chronological, interdisciplinary and informational dimensions.[107] These perspectives are in line with the NSF for Older People's principle of 'person-centred care' and this is the basic underlying principle of palliative care.

---

## Summary

- Deciding where the boundary lies between general elderly care and palliative care is problematic due to high levels of life-threatening co-morbidities.

- Elderly people are less likely to be referred for specialist palliative care.

- Non-cancer diagnoses with uncertain illness trajectories are common in elderly patients, making planning difficult.

- Multiple relocations from home to hospital and nursing home are not uncommon and often poorly planned.

- Continuity requires particularly well coordinated clinical and social service provision.

- The Single Assessment Process (SAP) is an attempt to ensure continuity for elderly patients.

---

## REFERENCES

1.  Davies E and Higginson IJ (eds). *Better Palliative Care for Older People*. Copenhagen: World Health Organization, 2004.

2.  Naylor MD. Transitional care of older adults. *Annual Review of Nursing Research* 2002; **20**: 127–47.

3.  Sturmberg JP and Schattner P. Personal doctoring. Its impact on continuity of care as measured by the comprehensiveness of care score. *Australian Family Physician* 2001; **30**: 513–18.

4.  Zarle NC. Continuity of care: Balancing care of elders between health care settings. *Nursing Clinics of North America* 1989; **24**: 697–705.

5.  Gill J. Can hospitalisations be avoided by having a regular source of care? *Family Medicine* 1997; **29**: 166–71.

6.  Kassa T, Loomis J, Gillis K, *et al*. The Edmonton Functional Assessment Tool: Preliminary development and evaluation for use in palliative care. *Journal of Pain and Symptom Management* 1997; **13**: 10–19.

7.  Wall E. Continuity of care and family medicine: Definition, determinants and relationship to outcome. *Journal of Family Practice* 1981; **13**: 755–64.

8.  McNeil C, Britton S, Nieuwendijk N and Rasmussen K. Closure of an in-hospital palliative home care service. *Journal of Palliative Care* 1998; **14**: 84–90.

9.  Hunt L. Continuity of care maximises autonomy of the elderly. *The American Journal of Occupational Therapy* 1998; **42**: 391–3.

10. Scholte op Reimer WJM, de Haan RJ, Limburg M and van den Bos GAM. Patients' satisfaction with care after stroke: Relation with characteristics of patients and care. *Quality in Health Care* 1996; **5**: 144–50.

11. Athlin E and Norberg A. Interaction between patients with severe dementia and their caregivers during feeding in a task-assignment versus a patient-assignment care system. *European Nurse* 1998; **3**: 215–27.

12. Cree M, Yang Q, Sclater A, *et al*. Continuity of care and health decline associated with a hip fracture. *Journal of Aging and Health* 2002; **14**: 385–98.

13. Jackson B, Hicks LE and Laughlin J. Bridge of continuity from hospital to nursing home – part 1: A proactive approach to reduce relocation stress syndrome in the elderly. *Continuum* 2000; **20**: 3–14.

14. Department of Health. *National Service Framework for Older People*. London: Department of Health, 2001.

15. Berkman B, Walker S, Bonander E and Holmes W. Early unplanned readmissions to social work of elderly patients: Factors predicting who needs follow-up services. *Social Work in Health Care* 1992; **17**: 103–19.

16. Magilvy JK and Lakomy JM. Transitions of older adults to home care. *Home Health Care Services Quarterly* 1991; **12**: 59–70.

17. Schultz A A, Geary P A, Casey F S and Fournier M A. Joining education and service in exploring discharge needs. *Journal of Community Health Nursing* 1997; **14**: 141–53.

18. Koroknay V. Collaborating for our patients' well-being. *Journal of Gerontological Nursing* 1997; **23**: 3–4.

19. Deutsch A and Neal J. National consensus conference on improving the continuum of care for patients with hip fracture. *Rehabilitation Nursing* 2002; **27**: 83–8.

20. Black D. King's fund care services enquiry. *Geriatric Medicine* 2004; **34**: 7.

21. Schonwetter R, Redmond L, Lowell J, *et al.* Palliative care. *Clinical Cardiology* 2000; **23**: S2 21–5.

22. Wennberg J E, Fisher E S, Stukel T A, *et al.* Use of hospitals, physician visits, and hospice care during last six months of life among cohorts loyal to highly respected hospitals in the United States. *British Medical Journal* 2004; **328**: 607–10.

23. Carline J D, Curtis R, Wenrich M D, *et al.* Physicians' interactions with health care teams and systems in the care of dying patients: Perspectives of dying patients, family members and health care professionals. *Journal of Pain and Symptom Management* 2003; **25**: 19–28.

24. Buxton V. Freedom of choice. *Nursing Times* 1996; **92**: 57–9.

25. McConnell E S. Preference for place of death in a continuing care retirement community. *The Gerontologist* 2001; **41**: 123–8.

26. Gallup Poll. Nationwide Gallup survey conducted for NHO in autumn 1996.

27. Gott M, Seymour J, Bellamy G, Clark D, Ahmedzai S H. Older people's views about home as a place of care at the end of life. *Palliative Medicine* 2004; **18 (5)**: 460–7.

28. Froggatt K. Life and death in English nursing homes: Sequestration or transition. *Ageing and Society* 2001; **21**: 319–32.

29. Catt S, Blanchard M, Addington-Hall J, Zis M, Blizard R and King M. Older adults' attitudes to death, palliative treatment and hospice care. *Palliative Medicine* 2005; **19**: 402–10.

30. Johnston G and Burge F. Analytic framework for clinician provision of end-of-life care. *Journal of Palliative Care* 2002; **18**: 141–9.

31. Skillbeck J, Mott L, Page H, Smith D, Ahmedzai S H and Clark D. Palliative care in chronic obstructive airways disease: A needs assessment. *Palliative Medicine* 1998; **12**: 245–54.

32. Gore J M, Brophy C J and Greenstone M A. How well do we care for patients with end-stage chronic obstructive pulmonary disease (COPD)? A comparison of palliative care and quality of life in COPD and lung cancer. *Thorax* 2000; **55**: 1000–6.

33. Edmonds P, Karlson S, Khan S and Addington-Hall J. A comparison of the palliative care needs of patients dying from chronical respiratory diseases and lung cancer. *Palliative Medicine* 2001; **15**: 287–95.

34. *The NHS and Community Care Act, 1990*. London: HMSO, 1990.

35. Cockram A, Gibb R and Kalra L. The role of a specialist team in implementing continuing health care guidelines in hospitalised patients. *Age and Ageing* 1997; **26**: 211–16.

36. The Continuing Care (NHS Responsibilities) Directions 2003.

37. West Midlands Strategic Health Authority. *NHS Responsibilities for Meeting Continuing Healthcare Needs and the NHS Contribution to Continuing Health and Social Care.* 2003.

38. Bull M J and Maruyama G M. Measuring continuity of elder's post hospital care. *Journal of Nursing Measurement* 2000; **8**: 41–60.

39. Singer P A and Bowman K W. Quality end-of-life care: A global perspective. *BMC Palliative Care* 2002; **1**: 4.

40. Finlay I. Dying with dignity. *Clinical Medicine* 2003; **3**: 102–3.

41. *Journal of the Royal College of Physicians of London.* The map of dying [editorial]. 2000; **34**: 325.

42. www.nice.org.uk/page.aspx?o=csgsp [accessed March 2007].

43. www.macmillan.org.uk [accessed March 2007].

44. www.cancerlancashire.org.uk [accessed March 2007].

45. www.lcp-mariecurie.org.uk [accessed March 2007].

46. Sahlberg-Blom E. The last month of life: Continuity, care site and place of death. *Palliative Medicine* 1998; **12**: 287–96.

47. Higginson I, Wade A and McCarthy M. Palliative care: Views of patients and their families. *British Medical Journal* 1990; **301 (6746)**: 277–81.

48. Vissner G, Klinkenberg M, Broese van Groenou M I, Willems D L, Knipscheer C P M and Deeg D J H. The end of life: Informal care for dying older people and its relationship to place of death. *Palliative Medicine* 2004; **18**: 468–77.

49. Wittenberg R, Pickard L, Comas-Herrera A, Davies B and Darton R. Demand for long-term care for older people in England to 2031. *National Statistics Quarterly* 2001; **12**: 5–16.

50. Burge F, Lawson B, Critchley P and Maxwell D. Transition in care during the end of life: Changes experienced following enrolment in a comprehensive palliative care program. *Palliative Care* 2005; **4**: 3.

51. Jackson M F. Use of community support services by elderly patients discharged from general medical and geriatric medical wards. *Journal of Advanced Nursing* 1990; **15**: 167–75.

52. Clare J and Hofmeyer A. Discharge planning and continuity of care for aged people: Indicators of satisfaction and implications for practice. *Australian Journal of Advanced Nursing* 1998; **16**: 7–13.

53. Jowett S and Armitage S. Hospital and community liaison links in nursing: The role of the liaison nurse. *Journal of Advanced Nursing* 1988; **13**: 579–87.

54. Anderson M and Helms L. Quality improvement in discharge planning: An evaluation of factors in communication between health care providers. *Journal of Nursing Care Quality* 1994; **8**: 62–72.

55. Victor C, Healy J, Thomas A and Seargent J. Older patients and delayed discharge from hospital. *Health and Social Care in the Community* 2001; **8**: 443.

56. Vetter N. Inappropriately delayed discharge from hospital: What do we know? *British Medical Journal* 2003; **326**: 927–8.

57. Murray S A, Boyd K, Kendall M, Worth A, *et al.* Dying of lung cancer or cardiac failure: Prospective qualitative interview study of patients and their carers in the community. *British Medical Journal* 2002; **325**: 929–34.

58. Murray S A, Kendall M, Boyd K and Sheikh A. Illness trajectories and palliative care. *British Medical Journal* 2005; **330**: 1007–11.

59. Higgs R. The diagnosis of dying. *Journal of the Royal College of Physicians of London* 1999; **33**: 110–12.

60. Iwasyna T and Christakis N. Attitude and self-reported practice regarding hospice referral in a national sample of internists. *Journal of Palliative Medicine* 1998; **1**: 241–8.

61. Hegney D, McCarthy A, de la Rue M B, Fahey P, *et al.* Discharge planning. *Collegian* 2002; **9**: 15–21.

62. Bowman C. The new imperative of long-term care. *Age and Ageing* 2002; **32**: 246–7.

63. Goodman C. Health needs in long term care. *Primary Health Care* 2003; **13**: 8.

64. Turnbull C. Community care – Are we moving forward? *Age and Ageing* 2001; **30**: 365–6.

65. Gillan J. Familiar problem. *Nursing Times* 1994; **90**: 54.

66. Wilber K H, Allen D, Shannon G R and Alongi S. Partnering managed care and community-based services for frail elders: The care advocated program. *Journal of the American Geriatrics Society* 2003; **51**: 807–12.

67. Caris-Verhallen W M C M and Kerkstra A. Continuity of care for patients on a waiting list for institutional long-term care. *Health and Social Care in the Community* 2001; **9**: 1–9.

68. www.hc-sc.gc.ca/seniors-aines/pubs/paho/paho_4_e.htm [accessed March 2007].

69. Reed J and Stanley D. Improving communication between hospitals and care homes: The development of a daily living plan for older people. *Health and Social Care in the Community* 2003; **11**: 356.

70. World Health Organization. *Cancer Pain Relief.* Geneva: WHO, 1996.

71. McGouran R C M. Dying with dignity. *Clinical Medicine* 2002; **2**: 43–4.

72. Huntington J. The proper contributors of social workers in health practice. *Social Science Medicine* 1986; **22**: 1151–60.

73. Toscani F, Borreani C, Boeri P and Miccinesi G. Life at the end of life: Beliefs about individual life after death and 'good death' models – a qualitative study. *Health and Quality of Life Outcomes* 2003; **1**: 65–75.

74. Saunders C. Into the valley of the shadow of death. A personal therapeutic journey. *British Medical Journal* 1996; **313**: 1599–1601.

75. Royal Commission on Long Term Care for the Elderly. Continuing Care Conference 1998.

76. Woodruff R. *Palliative Medicine: Symptomatic and supportive care for patients with advanced cancer and AIDS.* Melbourne: Oxford University Press, 1996.

77. Cox S. Improving communication between care settings. *Professional Nurse* 2000; **15**: 267–71.

78. Scott H. Research needed into the transfer of elderly people. *British Journal of Nursing* 1997; **6**: 844.

79. www.dh.gov.uk/PolicyAndGuidance/HealthAndSocialCareTopics/ SocialCare/SingleAssessmentProcess/fs/en [accessed March 2007].

80. Holland D E, Hansen D C, Matt-Hensrud N N, Severson M A, *et al.* Continuity of care: A nursing needs assessment instrument. *Geriatric Nursing* 1998; **19**: 331–4.

81. www.health.nsw.gov.au/ [accessed March 2007].

82. Dellasega C. Home alone. *Journal of Gerontological Nursing* 1992; **18**: 4.

83. Clough A. Community care policy and end-of-life care: One patient's story. *British Journal of Community Nursing* 2002; **7**: 153–7.

84. McDevitt J. A continuum of palliative care. *Canadian Nurse* 1992; **88**: 39–41.

85. Tichawa U. Creating a continuum of care for elderly individuals. *Journal of Gerontological Nursing* 2002; **28**: 46–52.

86. Payne S, Kerr C, Hawker S, Hardey M and Powell J. The Communication of information about older people between health and social care practitioners. *Age and Ageing* 2003; **31**: 107–17.

87. Pugh L C, Tringali R A, Boehmer J, Blaha C, *et al.* Partners in care: A model of collaboration. *Holistic Nursing Practice* 1999; **13**: 61–5.

88. Bull M J, Hansen H E and Gross C R. Differences in family caregiver outcomes by their level of involvement in discharge planning. *Applied Nursing Research* 2000; **13**: 76–82.

89. Bull M J, Hansen H E and Gross C R. A professional–patient partnership model of discharge planning with elders hospitalised with heart failure. *Applied Nursing Research* 2000; **13**: 19–28.

90. Addington-Hall J M. *Reaching Out: Specialist palliative care for adults with non-malignant diseases.* London: National Council for Hospices and Specialist Palliative Care Services and Scottish Partnership Agency, 1998.

91. Higginson I and Addington-Hall J M. *Palliative Care for Non-cancer Patients.* Oxford: Oxford University Press, 2001.

92. Barclay S, Todd C J, Grande G and Lipscombe J. How common is medical training in palliative care? A postal survey of general practitioners. *British Journal of General Practice* 1997; **47**: 800–5.

93. Street A and Blackford J. Communication issues for the interdisciplinary community palliative care team. *Journal of Clinical Nursing* 2001; **10**: 643–50.

94. Stahl L. How to transfer patients to other units. *American Journal of Nursing* 1996; **96**: 57–8.

95. Tellis-Nayak M. Understanding your patient's options. *American Journal of Nursing* 1998; **98**: 44–9.

96. Netten A, Darton R and Williams J. Nursing home closures: Effects on capacity and reasons for closure. *Age and Ageing* 2003; **32**: 332–7.

97. Darby P W. Quick response teams: A new approach in utilisation management. *Leadership in Health Services* 1992; **1**: 27–31.

98. von Sternberg T, Hepburn K, Cibuzar P, Convery L, *et al*. Post-hospital sub-acute care: An example of a managed care model. *Journal of the American Geriatrics Society* 1997; **45**: 87–91.

99. McNeil C, Britton S, Nieuwendijk N and Rasmussen K. Closure of an in-hospital palliative home care service. *Journal of Palliative Care* 1998; **14**: 84–90.

100. Abrahams R, Macko P and Grais M J. Across the great divide. *Journal of Case Management* 1992; **1**: 124–34.

101. Guttman R. Case management of the frail elderly in the community. *Clinical Nurse Specialist* 1999; **13**: 174–81.

102. Challis D, Darton R, Hughes J, Stewart K, *et al*. Intensive care-management at home: An alternative to institutional care? *Age and Ageing* 2001; **30**: 409–13.

103. Bailey M L. Care coordination in managed care creating a quality continuum for high risk elderly patients. *Nursing Case Management* 1998; **3**: 172–80.

104. Howarth G and Willison K. Preventing crises in palliative care in the home: The role of family physicians and nurses. *Canadian Family Physician* 1995; **41**: 439–45.

105. Mollica R. Coordinating services across the continuum of health, housing and supportive services. *Journal of Aging and Health* 2003; **15**: 165–88.

106. The Elderly Housing Coalition. Toward a national continuum of care. *Health Progress* 2000; **81**: 34–9.

107. McWhinney I R, Bass M J and Orr V. Factors associated with location of death (home or hospital) of patients referred to a palliative care team. *Canadian Medical Association Journal* 1995; **152**: 361–7.

108. Hennen B K D. Continuity of care in family practice, part 1: dimensions of continuity. *Journal of Family Practice* 1975; **2**: 371.

109. Wall E. Continuity of care and family medicine: Definition, determinants and relationship to outcome. *Journal of Family Practice* 1981; **13**: 755–64.

CHAPTER | 8

# Continuity of palliative care for people with non-malignant disease

*Angie Rogers, J. Simon R. Gibbs and Julia Addington-Hall*

## Introduction

In the United Kingdom, hospice and specialist palliative care has historically been associated with the care of cancer patients. However, as early as 1963 Hinton recognised that patients dying from non-malignant diseases were just as likely as cancer patients to experience distressing symptoms but were less likely to have them relieved.[1] A growing number of more recent research studies have highlighted the unmet health and social care needs of patients dying from non-malignant conditions,[2,3] while a number of government policy documents, most notably the National Service Frameworks for Coronary Disease and Long-Term Conditions, have acknowledged the need for palliative care among non-cancer patients.[4,5] The National Council for Palliative Care (NCPC) has published and supported both research and developmental work in this area.[6,7] However, the increased recognition of unmet needs among those dying from non-malignant conditions has yet to improve provision for these patients. The 2003–4 Minimum Data Set held by the NCPC indicated that between 5 and 6 per cent of new patients admitted to specialist palliative care in-patient facilities had a non-cancer diagnosis, with non-cancer patients accounting for 8 per cent of new day care patients, 5 per cent of new home care patients and 11 per cent of patients receiving support from a hospital-based specialist palliative care service.[8]

A number of reasons have been cited to account for such low numbers of non-cancer patients being cared for by specialists in palliative care. There may be a general reluctance on the part of palliative care specialists to become involved in the care of patients with non-malignant conditions as there is little available evidence as to what would constitute best clinical care, best practice or best service delivery for these patients. The diversity of presenting physical, emotional and social problems may be challenging to those with considerable expertise in caring for patients with cancer. There are difficulties associated with prognostication among patients dying from non-malignant conditions[9] and the disease trajectory, unlike that of the dying cancer patient, is likely to be characterised by acute deteriorations and partial recoveries.[10] These two factors have led to fears about palliative care services being overwhelmed not only by the sheer number of potential non-cancer referrals but also the long-term nursing needs of these patients.[11] Additionally, many independently funded hospices have raised funds specifically to care for cancer patients and may legally be unable or feel unable to provide services to other patients.

George and Sykes have suggested three different levels of input from specialists in palliative care. The first is short-term, focused consultations that might not necessarily be with the patients themselves, but with those caring for them, and will deal with discrete problems associated with pain and/or symptom management. The second is the full multidisciplinary support offered to cancer patients that might include in-patient, day and home care over a considerable period of time from a number of care providers. The third level is terminal care or care provided in the final days of life. This may be quite intensive but, again, the specialist in palliative care may more usually be acting in an advisory capacity to other healthcare professionals rather than providing care directly to the patient. The authors claim that the 'immediate logic of this approach is that it brings specialist palliative care into line with other specialties, namely that the fact, level and nature of advice or involvement is based on need rather than diagnosis'.[12] These models may have much to offer when considering the role of specialist palliative care in caring for patients dying from non-malignant conditions. Specialist palliative care expertise might be used to complement that of specialists working in other disciplines when problems arise with pain and or symptom management, or when intensive levels of terminal care are required. Alternatively, levels of need for some patients with non-malignant conditions may necessitate multidisciplinary input from a specialist palliative care team over a sustained period of time.

Most patients dying from non-malignant conditions will have been cared for, some for a considerable period of time, by their family doctors and hospital-based specialist, who may be reluctant to refer these patients to specialist palliative care services. There may be many reasons for this: clinicians may not wish to distress patients (or themselves) by talking about a patient's prognosis; they may not know which palliative care services are available; or, alternatively, they may feel competent to care for these patients without redress to specialist input. In terms of providing continuity of care some physicians may be reluctant to 'hand over' care of these patients at this point in the patient's illness. The majority of palliative care is provided within the community setting and GPs, district and specialist nurses, and other community-based professionals play a central role in caring for patients with non-malignant conditions.[13,14] As such, providing optimum palliative care for patients with non-malignant conditions relies not only on direct care from specialists in palliative care (which is likely to play a marginal role, at least at present) but also on the provision of advice and support from specialists in palliative care, and education in its principles and techniques for other health professionals.

The next section discusses some of the problems faced in providing continuing care for patients with non-malignant conditions who have palliative care needs and highlights a number of policy and developmental initiatives that may impact on continuity for this group of patients.

## Continuity of care

In a recent review of academic and policy literature Haggerty *et al.* identified three types of continuity that affect both patients' experiences and health professionals' perceptions of continuity of care.[15] These were discussed in Chapter 1.

These three types of continuity, informational, management and relational, personal or longitudinal, are useful when considering the continuity of care provided to people living with chronic illnesses or non-malignant conditions. However, toward the end of life when

---

Box 8.1 **Palliative care in non-malignant conditions**

- Hospice and specialist palliative care has to date been associated with the care of cancer patients.

- There is a growing body of evidence to indicate that patients dying from non-malignant conditions have unmet health and social needs.

- Symptom burden for patients dying from non-malignant conditions may be both longer lasting and more intense than for many cancer patients.

- Specialists in palliative care may be reluctant to care for patients with non-malignant conditions because of concerns about lack of personal expertise and/or the absence of an evidence base relating to effective treatments.

- Hospices and specialist palliative care services may be reluctant to take on these patients due to uncertainty about prognosis and fears of services being overwhelmed.

- Specialist palliative care involvement in non-malignant conditions may take the form of brief symptom-focused consultation, full multidisciplinary palliative care input as currently offered to many cancer patients, or terminal care, that is care in the last few days of life.

---

palliative care needs emerge a fourth dimension of continuity also comes into play: continuity in place of care. Place or location of care is especially important when considering the provision of palliative care. There is evidence to suggest that a dying patient's place of care often changes in the months, weeks and days leading to his or her death. Such changes in location of care will by necessity also be accompanied by changes in care providers and increase the potential for discontinuity in both management aims and informational continuity.[16] Additionally, changes in location of care may change the type of care offered to patients. In the acute hospital setting, treatments and interventions are predominately cure orientated, while in the hospice or other community setting provision more likely to be care orientated.

Continuity of care has a number of dimensions and while personal continuity may be desirable for both patients and practitioners other forms of continuity have arisen as the provision of health care has become more complex. However, it is perhaps the patients' and providers' experience of continuity that is most important. Haggerty *et al.* conclude:

For patients and their families, the experience of continuity is the perception that providers know what has happened before, that different providers agree on a management plan, and that a provider who knows them will care for them in the future. For providers, experience of continuity relates to their perception that they have sufficient knowledge and information about a patient to best apply their professional competence and the confidence that their care inputs will be recognised and pursued by other providers.[15]

Continuity of care may be more important to patients with chronic or severe illness as they are more likely to be seen by a number of healthcare providers, within different care locations and their health and social needs are likely to change rapidly.[17] However, changes in the provision of primary care described in Chapter 2 may decrease the chances of a patient being seen by the same doctor in the community setting,[18] and within the acute setting patients are likely to see a large number of healthcare providers, especially toward the end of life.[19] However, it is exactly these patients that are most likely to value continuity. As Weatherall states:

> Above all else those with distressing chronic or terminal illnesses need continuity of care – that is the attention and friendship of one doctor whom they can come to trust and with whom they can share their hopes and fears, yet this type of relationship is rarely available to them.[20]

## Continuity of care and non-malignant disease: the case of chronic heart failure

The research literature indicates that issues relating to uncertainty, complex therapeutic regimens, loss of physical functioning, poor psychological health and difficulties in obtaining information regarding their disease and its likely course are all common patient experiences. This is especially so among people with long-term chronic and/or life-limiting illnesses such as chronic heart failure. This section briefly outlines the literature on the experience of living with chronic heart failure and the impact the disease process and trajectory has upon the provision of care. It draws out issues relating to continuity of care

---

**Box 8.2  Continuity of care for people dying from non-malignant conditions**

A number of aspects of continuity are important in the provision of care for people dying from non-malignant conditions:

- Personal continuity occurs when one clinician is responsible for a patient over a period of time or a number of illness episodes. This type of continuity is valued by patients and clinicians but does not necessarily ensure that patients receive the most appropriate care or treatment.

- Continuity of aims of care achieved by open acknowledgement of patients' wishes, condition and likely prognosis, by all those caring for the patient and within the context of effective treatments and available services.

- Continuity of place of care achieved by limiting the number of changes in places of care for patients.

- Continuity achieved through the successful transfer of information between carer providers and between care providers and patients.

- Continuity achieved by adequate coordination of services and staff.

Each of these factors impacts on the others and therefore continuity of care.

---

that may be important for this group of patients in particular and non-cancer patients in general.

Heart failure is mainly a disease of old age with an estimated prevalence of 80.5 per 1000 population among those aged over 65 years. In the UK heart failure is thought to account for about 60,000 deaths per year.[21] Treatments for heart failure slow but do not arrest the progressive deterioration of myocardial function. Modern treatments rely on complex drug regimens that can include the use of angiotensin-converting enzyme inhibitors, angiotensin receptor blockers, beta-blockers and diuretics, with some patients also taking digoxin, aspirin, warfarin and anti-arrhythmic agents. Biventricular pacing and internal defibrillators are finding an increasing role. Additionally, patients may need to make changes to their diet, level of fluid intake and to adapt everyday routines to accommodate decreasing physical ability. Patients are also likely to be receiving medical treatments for other co-morbid conditions,[12,22] which may worsen their heart failure.[13]

Quality of life for these patients is known to be poor,[23] compromised psychological functioning often having a more significant impact than reduced physical ability.[24,25] Up to a third of these patients have been shown to have a major depression; depression is more common among patients with severe illness, impaired functional status and co-morbid psychiatric disorders; less than half of depressed patients receive any treatment at all for their depression.[26]

It can be seen that patients with chronic heart failure are likely to present with complex medical, psychological and social needs. As such they need individual tailored care, provided by someone with good background knowledge of the patient and his or her social setting or the ability to ascertain this quickly. A recent study of patients with chronic obstructive pulmonary disease (like heart failure, associated with increasing morbidity and a poor prognosis) indicated that patients' carers appreciate regular contact with a member of their primary care team for reassurance about the patient's condition. Contact with hospital-based clinics, however, were not valued in the same way, nor was the potential of a specialist nurse who the carers were likely to see as 'another stranger' or individual involved in their loved ones' care.[27] These patients and their carers valued personal or longitudinal continuity: not having to explain their story or their illness multiple times; and access to someone who was able to acknowledge their losses, with whom they could build an ongoing, trusting relationship. Clinically such a relationship may be important as it allows healthcare professionals to gauge what is 'normal' for an individual patient and hence be aware of when it is appropriate to adjust his or her medication or dietary restrictions and when to arrange an in-patient admission.

Most of the last year of life for patients with non-cancer is spent at home or in a nursing home under the care of the primary care team; however, many patients will have several episodes of hospital care within this time and the majority will go on to die within the acute hospital setting. Thus personal or longitudinal continuity provided by the primary care team will often be interrupted for patients with non-malignant conditions.

As with many other non-cancer conditions heart failure is characterised by periods of stability with acute exacerbations. Increased fluid retention results in symptomatic deterioration and hospital admission. Such episodes are often unexpected and in-patient care may be prolonged. However, patients can make near-full recoveries, and levels of physical functioning at the end of such admissions may be similar to or higher than those they had preceding such events.[28] Reported readmission rates are between 29 per cent and 46 per cent at three months and 36 per cent and 44 per cent at six months.[29] Such unplanned and frequent hospital admissions bring about inevitable changes in both the place of care and in care personnel, and may be accompanied by changes in the aims of care. The emphasis at present in heart failure is on acute exacerbations being managed by clinicians in hospitals rather than by GPs within the community. This highlights the need for informational continuity between primary and secondary care providers and between healthcare professionals and patients. It also provides an opportunity for heart failure nurse-led teams working across the primary–secondary care divide to provide care for patients regardless of whether they are in hospital or at home.

To date patients with heart failure have had little access to hospice-based palliative care but are increasingly seen by hospital-based palliative care teams and specialist heart failure nurses. However, whether this improves palliative care outcomes remains to be demonstrated.

**Challenges to continuity of palliative care**

Prognostication is difficult in heart failure; this is in part due to the risk of sudden death among patients with less severe heart failure and relatively stable symptoms. In New York Heart Association (NYHA) functional class II, symptoms are mild and annual mortality is reported to be between 5 and 15 per cent, with between 50 to 80 per cent of deaths being sudden.[30] In NYHA functional class IV, annual mortality is 30 to 70 per cent with only 5 to 30 per cent of deaths being sudden.[31] The relatively high risk of sudden death and high overall mortality rate make it difficult to determine when a patient is likely to die. Additionally, it is difficult to withdraw most active treatments for heart failure as such treatments play an important role in symptom relief. Recent research with heart failure patients has shown that many patients rarely think about dying or their own death in the context of their disease, other than during acute exacerbations.[32] These factors coupled with the acknowledged reluctance of doctors to discuss prognosis with patients and their families[33] hamper open communication regarding the disease, its trajectory and likely manner of death.

Perhaps the greatest inhibitor to continuity of care towards the end of life for chronic heart failure patients and those with other non-malignant conditions is the difficulty in making prognostic judgements, which prohibit the open acknowledgement by all parties that the patient's illness will lead inevitably to his or her death. Without such acknowledgement it is difficult to know what patients' wishes for end-of-life care are and impossible to plan for these. The use of scenario planning, when patients and their families are encouraged to consider three outcomes in terms of prognosis (short-term, medium-term and longer-term scenarios), as advocated by Dunlop,[34] may be useful in helping to ensure that care provided is consistent with that desired by patients and their carers. If patients do not want to think about their impending death it may be unethical for healthcare professionals to pursue such conversations. However, many patients have reported welcoming the chance to discuss their prognosis and likely manner of death, and perhaps best practice might be to provide adequate openings for patients to either initiate or pursue such conversations.

## Moving forward

The government currently advocates a system of case management for people with complex long-term conditions and/or high-intensity needs seeing community matrons as having a key role in coordinating care for these patients, ensuring successful transfer of information between providers and acting as the patients' advocate.[35] Despite its emphasis on reducing both hospital admissions and the length of hospital stays, case management could potentially enhance personal and informational continuity. Such personalised care plans would be developed in consultation with the patient, carers, relatives, health and social care professionals, based on a full assessment of medical, nursing and care needs. The plan would include preventative measures and anticipate future needs. Community matrons would be able to maintain contact with patients during hospital stays and to bring in additional support as needed from home, intermediate or pallia-

---

Box 8.3 **Chronic heart failure**

---

In common with many other non-malignant conditions:

■ Heart failure is a common chronic disease that leads to disability and death. Quality of life is often poor and symptom burden is greater than in some cancers. Modern treatments slow but do not halt the progression of the disease.

■ The successful management of heart failure relies on adherence to complex medical regimens, attention to dietary and fluid intake, and weight changes.

■ Heart failure is characterised by acute decompensations in heart and lung function, and is associated with frequent, unplanned hospital admissions and subsequent invasive treatments.

■ Research to date has shown that clinicians are reluctant to discuss the nature of these patients' diseases and inevitable outcomes, and patients are unlikely to have been told they are dying. However, many are thought to have worked this out for themselves and may welcome the opportunity to discuss this.

■ To date patients with heart failure have had little access to hospice-based palliative care but are increasingly seen by hospital-based palliative care teams and specialist heart failure nurses.

---

tive care teams. Specialist nurse practitioners for various disease groups including heart failure and chronic obstructive pulmonary disease (COPD) may fulfil a similar organisational and management role as community matrons, and provide the personal continuity valued by patients and their carers. In heart failure the provision of specialist nurses has been shown to reduce the number of hospital admissions for both heart failure and all causes, thus enhancing all four types of continuity.[36]

The majority of specialist heart failure nurses have a professional background in acute cardiology and may not be familiar with addressing the palliative care needs of their patients. As such they are likely to need training in generic palliative care, especially in being able to discuss end-of-life issues, the use of palliative medication and awareness of palliative care services and support. Once trained such nurses should be able to meet the palliative care needs of the vast majority of heart failure patients.[37]

Patients discharged from hospital may have had changes made

to their drug treatments, while their level of physical functioning may have changed. Additionally care needs and indeed those of their carer may have changed. As such patients may be particularly vulnerable at these times and adequate coordination of services and exchange of information will help ensure continuity of care.

In the absence of a community matron or specialist nurses a central repository such as NHS Direct for care plans may help ensure continuity of care aims and potentially place of care for patients with acute decompensations. However, issues relating to patient confidentiality and data protection would need to be addressed. Schemes that aim to inform out-of-hours primary care providers of palliative care patients may also enhance continuity of care.

Given that older people and those with more complex needs are likely to spend longer than four hours in accident and emergency departments prior to admission and that nursing staff report lacking the specialist skills to deal with vulnerable older people[38] the use of Integrated Care Pathways may have a positive impact on continuity for this group of patients. Such documents may be an important tool for bringing together past and current care, and for arranging for future needs; they may enhance best clinical practice and acknowledge social care needs. However, care pathways need to be flexible and to accommodate changes in patients' needs and circumstances. Patient-held plans may contribute to continuity of long-term care aims and can reduce the need for repeated case histories on the part of the patient and paperwork for healthcare professionals.[39]

The Liverpool Care Pathway offers a way of aiding the provision of evidence-based care to patients in their last days of life. Although developed to improve hospital-based care of dying cancer patients it has been successfully used in an acute stroke unit and at present a pathway for patients with heart failure is being developed.[40,41]

## Conclusion

Increased recognition of unmet health and social care needs among people dying from non-malignant conditions has yet to result in improved provision of services for this group. Several factors contribute to this: the general reluctance of specialist palliative care providers to take on the provision of care to this group; the lack of clear evidence on how best to manage these patients at the end of life; and the failure of government to identify additional or specific funding. Continuity of care is valued by both patients and healthcare professionals, and has undoubtedly been an important aspect of the provision of specialist palliative care to date.

In order to plan for the final phase of life, patients and their carers (both lay and professional) must know when they have or when they are likely to enter this phase. Clinicians report finding prognostication for patients with non-malignant disease difficult but may find it easier to acknowledge that a patient is suffering from a condition from which they are likely to die. The use of short, medium and long-term scenario planning, as suggested by Dunlop, may overcome some of the difficulties experienced in planning care for patients with indeterminate prognosis. As with cancer patients, beginning to make plans for palliative care early in the course of an illness may help ensure that patients' wishes are respected and may contribute to continuity of care in terms of both the aims and location of care. At the least, patients need to know how their illness is likely to progress, the aims of different interventions and how these are likely to affect them, the quality of their life and that of their wider family and loved ones. As such the importance of timely and open communication with these patients cannot be overstressed.

The acute exacerbations of symptoms seen in many non-cancer conditions, evident in chronic heart failure, may necessitate many unplanned changes in the location of care. These include the transitions from home care to care in the acute hospital setting and from hospital to community-based care, thus precluding personal continuity of care in terms of one key professional carer or one healthcare team. Good interprofessional communication has a key role in ensuring continuity at the end of life for these patients when moving between the secondary and primary healthcare sectors. In the future both clinical nurse specialists and community matrons may play a key role in ensuring continuity of care aims in different care settings and in ensuring that care remains patient focused, as they stand to enhance both the coordination of care between settings and the quality of communication between healthcare professionals. The use of care plans and patient-held notes might also improve communication between healthcare professionals working in disparate locations.

Initiatives that aim to alert out-of-hours primary and community care services to the presence of palliative care patients have an important role in enhancing continuity of care.

Further research is needed to more fully understand the ways in which continuity and discontinuity of care impact on patients' experiences at the end of life and what elements of care constitute 'good' continuity of care for these patients. More information is needed regarding ways in which acute exacerbations might be managed within community-based care settings as this would help to reduce the number of changes in care setting and personnel, and thus help ensure some measure of continuity.

Further research is also needed to enhance physicians' ability to prognosticate accurately in non-malignant conditions and importantly to assess whether such enhanced prognostication results in improved end-of-life care for these patients. More accurate prognostication may increase non-cancer patients' access to specialist palliative care. Providers who may then be less concerned about becoming involved in caring for patients with a 'long' prognosis and more concerned with enhancing both the quality of life and death for those dying from non-cancer conditions.

---

## Summary

- Continuity in terms of place of care, care personnel and information are all important in the provision of care to those dying from non-malignant conditions.

- Open communication with patients and clear lines of communication between those delivering health and social care are essential for all patients but are especially so when caring for those with non-malignant conditions during and following acute episodes.

- A key worker or central repository for information is essential to achieve adequate coordination of services, delivery of appropriate care and maintaining care aims for people with non-malignant conditions. In the future, community matrons, specialist nurses and NHS Direct may provide this function.

- A quick and planned response to rapidly changing clinical and social conditions is essential especially during 'out-of-hours' hours.

- Further research is needed to assess which aspects of continuity most impact on care provided to those dying of non-malignant conditions. Research should also concentrate on discovering which models of care most enhance continuity and hence the patient's care.

## Acknowledgements

AR is grateful for the help and support of Anne Holden while writing this text.

### REFERENCES

1. Hinton JM. The physical and mental stress of the dying. *Quarterly Journal of Medicine* 1963; **32**: 1–21.

2. Exley C, Field D, Jones L and Stokes T. Palliative care in the community for cancer and end-stage cardiorespiratory disease: The views of patients, lay-carers and health professionals. *Palliative Medicine* 2005; **19**: 76–83.

3. Hockley JM, Dunlop RJ and Davies RJ. Survey of distressing symptoms in dying patients and their families in hospital and the response to a symptom control team. *British Medical Journal* 1988; **296**: 1715–17.

4. Department of Health. *National Service Framework for Coronary Heart Disease*. London: Department of Health, March 2000.

5. Department of Health Long Term Conditions NSF Team. *The National Service Framework for Long-Term Conditions*. London: Department of Health, March 2005.

6. National Council for Palliative Care. *Focus on Policy – Branching out*. London: National Council for Palliative Care, May 2005.

7. Addington-Hall JM. *Reaching Out. Report of the Joint NCHSPCS and Scottish Partnership Agency Working Party on Palliative Care for Patients with Non-malignant Disease*. London: National Council for Hospice and Specialist Palliative Care Services, 1997.

8. The National Council for Palliative Care. *National Survey of Patient Activity Data for Specialist Palliative Care Services. Full report 2003–2004*. London: National Council for Palliative Care, April 2005.

9. Lynn J, Harrell F, Cohn F, Wagner D, *et al.* Prognosis of seriously ill hospitalized patients on the days before death: Implications for patient care and public policy. *New Horizons* 1997; **5**: 56–61.

10. Gibbs J S R. Heart disease. In: Addington-Hall J M and Higginson I J, eds. *Palliative Care for Non-cancer Patients.* Oxford: Oxford University Press, 2001, pp. 30–43.

11. Addington-Hall J M. Extending palliative care to chronic conditions. *European Journal of Palliative Care* 2005; **12(2)**: 14–17.

12. George R J D and Sykes J. Beyond cancer. In: Clark D, Hockley J and Ahmedzai S, eds. *New Themes in Palliative Care.* Buckingham: Open University, 1997, pp. 239–54.

13. Burt J, Shipman C, Addington-Hall J M and White P. *Perspectives on Caring for Dying Peope in London.* London: King's Fund, 2005.

14. Shipman C, Levenson R and Gillam S. *Psychosocial Support for Dying People. What can Primary Care Trusts do?* London: King's Fund, 2002.

15. Haggerty J L, Reid R J, Freeman G K, Starfield B H, *et al.* Continuity of care: A multidisciplinary review. *British Medical Journal* 2003; **327**: 1219–21.

16. Sahlberg E, Ternestedt B M and Johansson J E. The last month of life: Continuity, care site and place of death. *Palliative Medicine* 1998; **12**: 287–96.

17. Breslau N. Continuity re-examined: Differential impact on satisfaction with medical care for disabled and normal children. *Medical Care* 1982; **20**: 347–60.

18. Stokes T, Tarrant C, Freeman G and Baker R. Continuity of care and the new GMS contract: A survey of general practitioners in England and Wales. *Quality in Primary Care* 2005; **13**: 25–9.

19. Smith S D M, Nicol K M, Devereux J and Cornbleet M A. Encounters with doctors: Quality and quantity. *Palliative Medicine* 1999; **13**: 217–23.

20. Weatherall D J. The inhumanity of medicine. *British Medical Journal* 1994; **309**: 1671–72.

21. Cowie M R, Mosterd A, Wood D A, Deckers J W, *et al.* The epidemiology of heart failure. *European Heart Journal* 1997; **18**: 208–25.

22. Hakim R B, Teno J M, Harrell F E, Knaus W A, *et al.* Factors associated with do not resuscitate orders: Patients' preferences, prognoses, and physicians' judgements. SUPPORT investigators. Study to Understand Prognoses and Preferences for Outcomes and Risks of Treatments. *Annals of Internal Medicine* 1996; **125**: 284–93.

23. Stewart A L, Greenfield S, Hays R D, Wells K, *et al.* Functional status and well being of patients with chronic conditions. Results from a medical outcomes study. *Journal of the American Medical Association* 1989; **262**: 907–13.

24. Rideout E and Montemuro M. Hope, morale and adaptation in patients with chronic heart failure. *Journal of Advanced Nursing* 1986; **11**: 429–38.

25. Dracup K, Walden J A, Stevenson L W and Brecht M L. Quality of life in patients with advanced heart failure. *Journal of Heart and Lung Transplantation* 1992; **11**: 273–9.

26. Koenig H G. Depression in hospitalized older patients with congestive heart failure. *General Hospital Psychiatry* 1998; **20**: 29-43.

27. Seamark D A, Blake S D and Seamark C J. Living with severe chronic obstructive pulmonary disease (COPD): Perceptions of patients and their carers. *Palliative Medicine* 2004; **18**: 619–25.

28. Jaagosild P, Dawson N V, Thomas C, Wenger N S, *et al.* Outcomes of acute exacerbation of severe congestive heart failure: Quality of life, resource use, and survival. SUPPORT Investigators. The Study to Understand Prognosis and Preferences for Outcomes and Risks of Treatments. *Archives of Internal Medicine* 1998; **158**: 1081–9.

29. Rich M W, Beckham V, Wittenberg C, Leven C L, *et al.* A multidisciplinary intervention to prevent the readmission of elderly patients with congestive heart failure. *New England Journal of Medicine* 1995; **333**: 1190–5.

30. Kjekshus J. Arrhythmias and mortality from congestive heart failure. *American Journal of Cardiology* 1990; **65**: 421–81.

31. Califf R M, Adams K F, McKenna W J, Gheorghiade M, *et al.* A randomized control trial of epoprostenol therapy for severe congestive heart failure: The Flolan International Randomized Survival Trial (FIRST). *American Heart Journal* 1997; **134**: 44–54.

32. Willems DL, Hak A, Visser F and Van de Wal G. Thoughts of patients with advanced heart failure on dying. *Palliative Medicine* 2004; **18**: 564–72.

33. Elkington H, White P, Higgs R and Pettinari C J. GPs' views of discussions of prognosis in severe COPD. *Family Practice* 2001; **18**: 440–4.

34. Dunlop R. Specialist palliative care and non-malignant diseases. In: Addington-Hall J M and Higginson I J, eds. *Palliative Care for Non-cancer Patients*. Oxford: Oxford University Press, 2001, pp. 189–97.

35. Department of Health. *Supporting People with Long Term Conditions. Improving care. Improving lives*. London: Department of Health, January 2005.

36. Blue L, Long E, McMurray J, Davie A P, *et al.* Randomised controlled trial of specialist nurse intervention in heart failure. *British Medical Journal* 2001; **323**: 715–18.

37. Segal DI, O'Hanlon D, Rahman N, *et al.* Incorporating palliative care into heart failure management: A new model of care. *International Journal of Palliative Nursing* 2005; **11 (3)**: 135–6.

38. National Audit Office. *Improving Emergency Care in England. Report by the Comptroller and Auditor General*. London: The Stationery Office, October 2004.

39. Campbell H, Hotchkiss R, Bradshaw N and Porteous M. Integrated care pathways. *British Medical Journal* 1998; **316**: 133–7.

40. Ellershaw J and Wilkinson S. *Care of the Dying. A pathway to excellence*. Oxford: Oxford University Press, 2003.

41. National Council for Palliative Care. Information exchange. February 2005.

CHAPTER | 9

# Continuing spiritual care

*Edward Pogmore*

## Introduction

There has never been such an interest in the spiritual and religious needs of people. This is partly because of the multicultural diversity of British society and the rise of alternative spiritual experience at the start of a new millennium. Perhaps it is also due to the uncertain times in which we live when the technical and scientific solutions to our problems seem to have failed to live up to their previous promise.

When we attend the medical centre at times of illness, wait apprehensively in the doctor's 'out-of-hours' waiting room or find ourselves coming round in the A & E resus room, we are likely to ask the question 'Why is this happening to me?' This is a spiritual question. At such times we are likely to look for help from our own support systems, be they family, friends or our religious and non-religious communities. We are also likely to examine our own beliefs and world view, be they religious or philosophical. Whether or not we have a religious framework within which we start to work through such questions, these are none the less spiritual issues.

The central issues surrounding the spiritual needs of patients facing a serious and life-threatening illness have been recognised within hospice and palliative care from the earliest times. This has recently been formalised within the National Institute for Health and Clinical Excellence (NICE) *Guidance on Cancer Services: Improving supportive and palliative care for adults with cancer*. The section on spiritual support services states that:

> Beliefs can be religious, philosophical or broadly spiritual in nature. Formal religion is a means of expressing an underlying spirituality, but spiritual belief, concerned with the search for the existential or ultimate meaning in life, is a broader concept and may not always

be expressed in a religious way. It usually includes reference to a power other than self, often described as 'God', a 'higher power', or 'forces of nature'. This power is generally seen to help a person to transcend immediate experience and to re-establish hope.[1]

Spiritual care has not always been seen as a vital part of clinical care among the healthcare professions. In a survey of general practitioners, although most saw, in theory, a role for clergy in the areas of bereavement care, divorce, depression or chronic illness, this was generally unrealised in practice.[2] Whilst spiritual and religious care is included as part of mandatory training for doctors, its scope is narrow.[3] Nurses too, although they commonly consider providing spiritual support as an important aspect of their role, have reported a lack of knowledge and skills in providing such care.[4] In practice many healthcare professionals do express interest in receiving greater help and training in the process of assessing and meeting the spiritual needs of patients. Many clergy of all faith traditions (who work outside healthcare settings) also express the desire for more expertise in assessing health-related spiritual needs.

As the spiritual needs of patients are being personally articulated not necessarily in religious terms, those needs are becoming more sophisticated and diverse. Beliefs and practices of patients in modern society within the UK include those of the main religious faiths: Bahai, Buddhist, Christian, Hindu, Jain, Jewish, Muslim, Sikh, Zoroastrian, etc, but also other beliefs including Pagan, Humanist and New Age religions. Spiritual needs require appropriate responses from the whole healthcare team. This involves not merely an appreciation of the differences between different faiths, but also an awareness that variations between individuals exist even within these mainstream faiths.[5] It is important that healthcare professionals are aware of such denominational, cultural and indeed personal differences that need to be considered.

Modern hospices and palliative care services have a long association with spiritual and religious care. However, within Christian culture there is also a history of providing holistic care. The abbeys and priories of Britain and continental Europe bear witness to this tradition of hospitality and binding up the wounds of travellers. The origin of the word hospice takes us to these places – 'a traveller's place of rest'. The term 'palliative care' arising from the word *'palliare'* in Latin for 'cloak' includes the concept of covering all aspects of care, of which spiritual care and also religious care form part.

This chapter will relate to the individual needs of people and their families of all backgrounds and faith traditions including those whose 'faith' may be atheist or agnostic – and will offer a definition of what spiritual care encompasses. It will particularly focus on how continuity of care is a vital concept for the provision of spiritual care. Finally, the whole approach to palliative care 'open all hours' will be evaluated in the light of spiritual care developments and the associated educational and training needs.

## Spirituality in relation to palliative care

In considering spiritual care and in particular the issue of continuity, the following elements need to be considered.

- Spiritual care within palliative care cannot ever be narrow. Caring for the whole person includes attention to the environment and the context of care. The practical details that enable the appropriate context are vital. Wherever possible the person needs to be cared for in the environment of his or her choosing, an aspect that needs to be explored as part of an early, thorough and ongoing assessment, in order that the appropriate care can be given in and out of hours.

- Spiritual care of informal carers, both families and friends, and caring for the wider professional care team are also important aspects to be considered.

- Education within multidisciplinary teams is vital to the process of assessing spiritual need so that it becomes central to the assessment of a person's needs and is undertaken in an unselfconscious manner.

- In providing continuity of care the organisation of spiritual care in palliative care teams needs to be considered. The future developments of healthcare chaplaincy for all patients should work towards the integration of care between hospices, hospitals and primary care initiatives, so that a seamless service can be achieved. The role of cancer networks may be particularly important in these strategic developments.

Palliative care teams usually have chaplaincy input via a chaplain either in a part-time or full-time capacity. They should be available to advise staff regarding assessment of spiritual and religious needs, and to liaise with all faith leaders regarding appropriate community support.

'Out of hours' in the religious and spiritual context is a strange concept. All hours are religious and indeed spiritual. The patient and their carers may face a crisis and need support at any time of the day or night. This, however, needs to be balanced with the needs of professional care givers, including clergy, for time off duty. Within these constraints the organisation of religious and spiritual care needs to be approached in such a way as to be a natural aspect of holistic care, with continuity of professional availability being offered. Since personal continuity of one professional is impossible to achieve, briefing of colleagues, appropriate to the individual and the family needs, is a vital aspect of care. Clearly this should be made at an appropriate level, on a need-to-know basis, with the patient's understanding of the necessity for such briefing and their permission to such sharing within the team, so that confidentiality may be maintained.

**Defining spiritual care**

Numerous definitions of spiritual care exist in the literature. Lyall's definition suggests that it has the following characteristics.

'Spiritual care:

- Is a response to the spiritual needs of a person understood through exploring life events, beliefs, values and meaning.
- Is a means of therapeutic support to enable a person challenged by illness, trauma, or bereavement to find meaning in their experiences of vulnerability, loss or dislocation.
- Addresses the existential, transcendental, biographical and temporal dimensions of illness, disability, suffering and bereavement.

- Contributes to healing and rehabilitation in respecting the integrity of the person and by attending to wholeness in the midst of brokenness.
- May incorporate psychological, social and religious dimensions.'[6]

From the experience of practice this is a helpful start in pinning down the enormous diversity of individual responses to the experience of unease or disease. This definition is utilised in the document *Caring for the Spirit*, which outlines a practical model of spiritual care under the domains familiar to other disciplines within palliative care:

- assessment
- care planning
- care delivery
- continuous review.[7]

At its best spiritual care promotes and protects fundamental values of the person keeping these at the centre of his or her care, remembering that we are only involved as a result of his or her invitation to us.

In the seminal book *Mud and Stars* the 'concept of care' in the modern hospice is described.

Hospice seeks to prevent last days becoming lost days. It attempts to do this by offering a type of care which is appropriate to the needs of the dying. Although it has been described as 'low tech and high touch', hospice is not against modern medical technology. Rather it seeks to ensure that love and not science is the controlling force in patient care. 'High tech' investigations and treatments are used only when their benefits clearly outweigh any potential burdens. Thus, science is used in the service of love and not vice versa. In summary, hospice care is an attempt to re-establish the traditional role of doctors and other clinical staff.[8]

Care is given in the context of hope, which is one of the values that spiritual care endeavours to protect. Hope is not just wishing for something better, but a fundamental purpose that gives meaning to and purpose for the immediate moment and the building of trust for the future.

Hope is threatened when the patient is isolated by a 'conspiracy of silence', feeling abandoned by professional carers, suffering uncontrolled physical symptoms and unrecognised depression. Similarly a future seeming to offer nothing but an 'insuperable mountain of problems' and unaddressed spiritual distress are potent destroyers of hope.

The task of the carer is to restore hope displaying 'unconditional acceptance' of the patient through listening, addressing and relieving troublesome symptoms, establishing trust and enabling the patient to establish realistic goals. The distinct role of spiritual care is to offer companionship.[8]

The 2004 NICE Guidance on Supportive and Palliative Care points out that the needs of patients for spiritual support are frequently unrecognised by health and social care professionals, who may feel uncomfortable broaching spiritual issues. The Key Recommendation 11 suggests that:

> Patients and carers should have access to staff who are sensitive to their spiritual needs. Multidisciplinary teams should have access to suitably qualified, authorised and appointed spiritual care givers who can act as a resource for patients, carers and staff. They should also be aware of local community resources for spiritual care.

The guidelines stress that palliative care should be available 24 hours a day and spiritual care should be integral to that availability.

The central nature of spiritual care is stressed in a recent editorial by Speck, Higginson and Addington-Hall, who argue that

> Evidence is growing that spiritual belief and religious practice are important predictive factors for a larger proportion of people entering health care than previously thought. Many may benefit from support for this aspect of their life. A need exists for user friendly and brief measures to assess spiritual need in the absence of religious faith, so that it may be addressed properly rather than as some general panacea which is assumed to be good but is not individually tailored. Only in this way we 'ensure that the spiritual elements of disease are taken into account,' as recommended in the guidance from NICE.[9]

## Organising spiritual care in the palliative care team

Spiritual care needs to be organised in such a way that it is seamlessly integrated with care by the rest of the palliative care team. Such an approach will enable the patient to experience it as a natural part of the holistic approach. Spiritual aspects are best included within the patient's palliative care record, encouraging continuity as with any other area of care.

There is a wide variation in the organisational and workforce make-up of healthcare chaplaincy in the UK.[10] Palliative care teams, especially those attached to hospice units, usually have chaplaincy input via a chaplain either part time or full time. As well as having a face-to-face role, chaplains should also be available to advise staff regarding assessment of spiritual and religious needs. A vital part of their role is liaison with other faith leaders to provide religiously and culturally appropriate care for individual patients and also enabling appropriate community support. In many teams the chaplain will attend multidisciplinary team meetings and will be seen as an equal member of the team. Chaplaincy teams are often supported by volunteers who receive training in basic spiritual care, especially listening skills. These can provide valuable assistance in the provision of spiritual care, particularly in giving time to patients, their families and carers, and also the staff.

It is also important for members of the palliative care team to be aware of religious and spiritual needs of patients, and feel competent in responding to these and knowing to what extent they can participate in providing support. A framework for four levels of competency in providing spiritual care aimed at supporting staff and volunteers has been developed by the Marie Curie group of hospices. The competencies identify levels beyond which members of staff would not expect to proceed and give clear guidelines on when to refer to the chaplain or chaplaincy staff (see Box 9.1). Evaluation of a pilot study found that the approach affirmed good practice and that 'personal skills and limits are recognised, and training and development needs are identified'.[11]

In providing 24-hour care chaplains should be part of an 'on call' network of other chaplains who will be available to assess needs of individuals and families, provide support for patients, relatives and staff, and perform religious and ceremonial duties as appropriate.

---

Box 9.1 **Spiritual and religious competencies**

Level 1 is for all staff and volunteers who have casual contact with patients and their families. This level seeks to ensure that all staff and volunteers understand that all people have spiritual needs, and distinguishes spiritual and religious needs. It seeks to encourage basic skills of awareness, relationships and communication, and an ability to refer concerns to members of the multidisciplinary team.

Level 2 is for staff and volunteers whose duties require contact with patients and family/carers. This level seeks to enhance the competencies developed at level 1 with an increased awareness of spiritual and religious needs, and how they may be identified and responded to. In addition to increased communication skills, identification and referral of difficult needs should be achievable, along with an ability to identify personal training needs.

Level 3 is for staff and volunteers who are members of the multidisciplinary team. This level seeks to further enhance the skills of levels 1 and 2. It moves into the area of assessment of spiritual and religious need, developing a plan for care and recognising complex spiritual, religious and ethical issues. This level also introduces confidentiality and the recording of sensitive and personal patient information.

Level 4 is for staff or volunteers whose primary responsibility is for the spiritual and religious care of patients, visitors and staff. Staff working at level 4 are expected to be able to manage and facilitate complex spiritual and religious needs in patients, families/carers, staff and volunteers, in particular the existential and practical needs arising from the impact on individuals and families of issues in illness, life, dying and death. In addition, they should have a clear understanding of their own personal beliefs and be able to journey with others focused on the patient's needs and agendas. They should liaise with external personnel and access resources as required. They should also act as a resource for support, training and education of healthcare professionals and volunteers, and seek to be involved in professional and national initiatives.

---

*Source*: Gordon and Mitchell.[11]

Where this is not the case, very often it will be the local parish clergy, ministers and faith leaders who may have the natural connections with patients, and will be invariably willing to provide this continuity of care. Staff should know who to call and have access to appropriate contact telephone numbers. One model is to have a central PCT list that can be held by the primary care out-of-hours provider. All the major faiths should have designated leaders who can be contacted via the local hospital chaplain, who will keep an updated list of first-line contacts. The on-call chaplain should be able to contact such faith leaders at short notice out of hours.

For patients and carers who already have a local link with their church or faith centre, out-of-hours contact numbers will often be available. Sometimes the local church or faith centre will have a pastoral care team who share the responsibility of care and have an agreed local contact with families. The local 'Churches Together' [loose groupings of churches within an area, cooperating on local religious and spiritual issues] will normally also have up-to-date lists of Christian clergy and their contact numbers, which can be obtained through the main Christian ministers of the locality. Very often there are multi-faith organisations and intercultural groups that can supply information and advice about appropriate care. Many hospital trusts have multilingual support workers working closely with the Patient Advice and Liaison Service (PALS), who can aid in communicating with patients who are speakers of languages other than English.

**Elements of out-of-hours spiritual care**

Chaplains may be required to perform a number of specific tasks out of hours. Patients and carers require prayer at vulnerable times. This might be in the last hours of life, at the time of dying or prayers of commendation after death. In an emergency situation, prayers can even be said over the telephone to provide immediate support whilst personal contact is arranged as a follow-up. Sometimes it is the 'presence' of a chaplain that can provide support for patients and their families. At times the patient and family require an advocate to enable them to say sorry for past hurts when it is too painful to share them directly.

On some occasions the role of the chaplain is to provide practical help for the patient with regard to funeral arrangements or last wishes. It can be a request to help with arrangements to marry near to death, which includes liaison with the Registrar for Marriages out of hours. Chaplains often develop close working relationships with funeral directors and can help in facilitating arrangements, especially in circumstances where specific religious or cultural observances need to be made.

Acts of ceremony are important to many, especially immediately before or after death. Words from a specific liturgy, special prayers and various practical acts, for example communion, anointing, etc., which will vary between faiths and traditions, might all be necessary out of hours. Such activities may well need to be performed by ordained clergy from the appropriate denomination or faith tradition, whose contact details therefore should be recorded in advance.

If the faith tradition requires that a body is touched or prepared in a particular way following death, nursing staff should be aware of this to enable the appropriate action to be taken (see Box 9.2).

---

Box 9.2 **Examples of ceremonial aspects of different faiths at the time of death**

- Judaism – no last rites. Dying patients will sometimes ask for a rabbi, who will recite a prayer called the Shema. The body is placed on the floor with feet towards the door by the family. Normally the body is not moved on the Sabbath, although it is understood that this is not practical in hospitals or hospices.

- Sikhism – comfort at time of death may be given by readings from the Guru Granth Sahib and private prayers. After death the family will wash and dress the body. Cremation normally takes place as soon as possible after death.

- Hinduism – death is accepted as inevitable and rarely met with anger as in Judaism, Islam or Christianity. A Hindu priest (pandit) will often help the patient with his or her acts of worship. Customs do vary. Cremation takes place. The Ganges is the sacred river for cremations and Ganges water is often present at funerals.

- Islam – the presence of an imam is not required at the time of death but the family may whisper the call to prayer in the dying person's ear with the person's face towards Mecca. After death, the body should not be touched by a non-Muslim. If it needs to be, as in a hospital or hospice, gloves can prevent actual contact. Muslims are buried, not cremated, usually within 24 hours.

---

*Source*: Neuberger.[12]

Front-line staff working with dying patients often face distressing situations out of hours. Whilst a good death should be the aim of all care it is often difficult to achieve and the act of dying may be unpleasant or distressing. Staff may have formed close ties with a patient over a period of time and having to deal with their death in the context of continuing to care for other patients on a busy shift can be particularly difficult. Other stressful situations might include the death of a young person and dealing with distressed relatives or bereaved children. It is an important part of the chaplain's role to be involved in the care of such patients, sharing the burden with other staff, but also to provide support to the staff themselves.

## Summary of key aspects of continuity for spiritual care

*Good assessment* of spiritual and religious needs at the earliest possible stage by the primary caring team – i.e. district nurse or GP in the community and ward nurses for in-patients – should be made. The specialist palliative care team might also be involved in this process and the chaplain can offer general support and advice. Often the chaplain will be part of this assessment through direct contact with the patient, particularly if special needs are discovered by the primary caring team, but spiritual assessment is by no means the sole preserve of the chaplain. Competency tools to support healthcare staff in such assessments may foster greater confidence and involvement.

Ongoing spiritual needs and care should be reviewed as part of the multidisciplinary team process. This is partly an acknowledgement of tendency for spiritual insights from the patient to emerge slowly over time as relationships and openness in communication develop. Also it enables 'out of hours' care to be organised where possible ahead of time. Similarly if an unforeseen emergency occurs, such a review should facilitate accessing appropriate care by ensuring that specific instructions and contact numbers are available for the patient.

*Ensuring that personal continuity of care* is maintained is important, with the patient and family receiving care from a single chaplain or chaplaincy visitor as far as possible. Sometimes a partnership between the chaplain and the patient's own faith leader or minister will be appropriate to ensure ongoing and appropriate care. The presence of someone familiar, in whom trust has developed, can be particularly important at significant times, for example close to or after death or when bad news has been received. Whatever the arrangement for care it should be led by the patient and where that is not possible the closest family member who understands his or her needs and wishes.

*Education and liaison arrangements* are important so that local faith leaders know the general outline of the local palliative care approach and 'out of hours' arrangements. These relationships are so important for the building of local networks to ensure that care can be as integrated as possible. The Primary Care Trusts (PCTs) will usually build up a database of contacts in faith communities. In North Warwickshire as part of our integrated chaplaincy team for the NHS hospital trust and the PCT, we now employ a Community Development Chaplain whose brief, in part, is to develop personal links with all the faith communities (see Box 9.3). Particular attention needs to be paid in a situation where a patient is a member of a minority faith community with which links have not already been developed.

---

Box 9.3 **North Warwickshire integrated chaplaincy team**

- Team serving both hospital, PCT, Mental Health Partnership and hospice that provides palliative day care and hospice at home.
- Multi-denominational team including main Christian denominations and an imam, providing care for the large Muslim population in the area, and representatives from the Sikh and Hindu communities.
- Palliative care chaplain who is part of the multidisciplinary palliative care team and provides specific input for patients at the day hospice and receiving care through the Hospice at Home team and in the local hospital.
- Volunteer workers who receive training in spiritual care including listening and palliative care, working under the supervision of the chaplains.
- Community development chaplain builds and maintains links with clergy and faith leaders in the local community, and gives pastoral support to the local GPs and their staff.
- On-call rota of chaplains providing 24-hour care contactable via the local hospital switchboard and available to hospital, hospice and community staff.

---

*Spiritual care of the healthcare team* is an important aspect of the chaplain's work both in offering advice in spiritual assessment to develop skills and build confidence in this area, equipping them more fully to deliver holistic care, but also in offering support, encouragement and debriefing in and 'out of hours'.

## Postscript

At its best palliative care is practical, personal and responsive, and should be accessible at all times. The way we help people at the end of life and through death illustrates what value we have for life in general. The precious nature of life itself becomes very clear when we work with those who are dying.

In- and out-of-hours spiritual care needs to be adequately resourced, to give care that is vital and timely to the patient, the family and for the team who are working in one of the most sensitive and stretching parts of health care. Investment in out-of-hours spiritual care in the acute and primary care settings has been poor, which can have an adverse effect on quality. Spiritual care should be included within a quality and clinical governance framework, and should be taken as seriously as any other aspect of holistic care.

'Holy' and 'wholly' are close together in meaning. They express the uniqueness of each individual and the need to facilitate fullness of life until inevitable death. Spiritual care in all its diversity should be at the centre of that whole care.

### Acknowledgement

I am grateful to Rev. Prebendary Peter Speck for helpful comments on an earlier draft of this chapter.

---

## Summary

- Spiritual or existential issues are experienced by any patient facing death, not just the religious.

- Spiritual care should be offered as part of the multidisciplinary approach in palliative care.

- Continuity should be maintained by thorough assessment and planning to ensure appropriate spiritual help is available in and out of hours.

- The role of the chaplain is: providing support to patients and families; offering religious offices; liaising with local clergy and leaders from all faiths; and providing support and training for other healthcare staff.

- Religious and cultural differences should be understood and plans should be made for appropriate rituals to be performed as needed in or out of hours.

---

**USEFUL WEBSITES**

- www.healthcarechaplains.org □ the website of the College of Health Care Chaplains.

- www.hospitalchaplain.com □ a worldwide website concerning pastoral care for the healthcare chaplain.

- www.ahpcc.org.uk □ the website for the Association of Hospice and Palliative Care Chaplains.

- www.nhs-chaplaincy-spiritualcare.org.uk/ □ the website of the Hospital Chaplaincies Council.

- www.web-scribeuk.net/Spiritual-Needs □ a website specifically concerning people with learning disabilities.

- www.mfghc.com □ the website of the National Multi-Faith Group set up to advance multi-faith healthcare chaplaincy in England and Wales.

- www.sach.org.uk □ the website of the Scottish Association of Chaplains.

**REFERENCES**

1. *Guidance on Cancer Services: Improving supportive and palliative care for adults with cancer.* London: National Institute for Clinical Excellence, 2004.

2. Jones A. A survey of general practitioners' attitudes to the involvement of clergy in patient care. *British Journal of General Practice* 1990; **40**: 280–3.

3. *The New Doctor: Recommendations on general clinical training.* London: General Medical Council, 1997.

4. Kuuppelomaki M. Spiritual support for nursing terminally ill patients: Nursing staff assessments. *Journal of Clinical Nursing* 2001; **10**: 660–70.

5. Cobb M. Spiritual care. In: Lloyd-Williams M, ed. *Psychosocial Issues in Palliative Care.* Oxford: Oxford University Press, 2003, pp. 135–47.

6. Lyall D. *The Integrity of Pastoral Care* (New library of pastoral care). London: SPCK, 2001.

7. *Caring for the Spirit.* South Yorkshire Workforce Development Confederation, 2003.

8. *Mud and Stars: Working party on the impact of hospice experience on the Church's healing ministry.* Oxford: Sobell Publications, 1991.

9. Speck P, Higginson I and Addington-Hall J. Spiritual needs in healthcare. *British Medical Journal* 2004; **329**: 123–4.

10. Wright M. Chaplaincy in hospice and hospital: Findings from a survey in England and Wales. *Palliative Medicine* 2001; **15**: 229–42.

11. Gordon T and Mitchell D. A competency model for the assessment and delivery of spiritual care. *Palliative Medicine* 2004; **18**: 646–51.

12. Neuberger J. *Caring for Dying People of Different Faiths.* London: Mosby, 1994.

CHAPTER | 10

# PCTs and organisational issues in continuity of palliative care

*Jenni Burt and Gloria Jones*

## Introduction

Recent years have seen rapid changes in the organisational structures within which healthcare services are planned and secured. The provision of palliative care, both in and out of hours, is now assessed, planned and commissioned by Primary Care Trusts (PCTs), overseen by Cancer Networks. Unprecedented changes in the responsibilities of general practitioners – including the opt-out of 24-hour responsibility for their patients, the increasing responsibilities of the nursing profession, and the reorganisation of the provision of unplanned medical care – have created both exciting opportunities for the provision of innovative urgent care services, and the real fear that patients, especially vulnerable patients including those with palliative care needs, may fall 'through the net'. This chapter will consider issues in continuity of palliative care at the organisational level and examine recent developments and current proposals, many of which are yet to be fully defined, and all of which are likely to have wide-ranging effects on the delivery of health care. It first considers the responsibilities of PCTs in securing and delivering services within the 'commissioning cycle'. It then outlines the context for the provision of unscheduled care, and the new organisational structures that current policy is encouraging to take shape. The challenges of meeting the continuing care needs of palliative patients within the new organisational structures are then considered, with a consideration of concerns that must be addressed if patients are to receive the high-quality care they deserve.

## Roles, responsibilities and the organisation of services

During this decade, PCTs have emerged as the lead English NHS organisations in assessing need, planning and securing all health services and improving health in their localities.[1] It has been a rapid rise. There were just 17 PCTs in existence in April 2000[2] – and 303 by 2005. The process of evolution is continuing with further restructuring and mergers implemented by the Department of Health from 2006 as part of 'commissioning a patient-led NHS'.

Currently, PCTs hold over 75 per cent of the NHS budget, which they must spend in accordance with both local priorities and national targets. Alongside acute care, PCTs are also responsible for providing most community services and developing primary care services, including GPs and district and community nursing services – although this function may well reduce with the implementation of the government's plans to strengthen the commissioning role. Within palliative care, PCT functions currently include the following.

### Securing the provision of services

- Taking responsibility for the management, development and integration of all primary care services in the light of the changes set out in the NHS Plan and NHS Cancer Plan.[2,3] Commissioning all specialist cancer and palliative care services (community, secondary, tertiary and voluntary sector), in collaboration with other local PCTs and the Cancer and/or Supportive and Palliative Care Networks.

### Integrating health and social care

- Working with local authorities to integrate health and social care (through the use of the Health Act flexibilities and through the use of the Health and Social Care Act 2001 and the wellbeing power in the Local Government Act 2000), to help ensure integrated and fast-tracked services for cancer and palliative care patients receiving care at home.

However, palliative care is seldom a priority for PCTs, faced as they are with an array of other, key, 'must-do's' set out by the government. A workshop on commissioning held by Help the Hospices in December 2002 found that, in order to gain attention at PCT level, palliative care was most profitably linked with imperatives such as the National Service Framework for Older People.[4] This provided the necessary impetus for PCTs to take action. Such an impetus has also been provided by the £50 million allocated to specialist palliative care services, and the publication of the National Institute for Health and Clinical Excellence (NICE) *Guidance on Cancer Services: Improving supportive and specialist palliative care for adults with cancer.*[5]

A further challenge for the coordination and provision of palliative care for PCTs is the complexity of existing palliative care provision that PCTs have inherited.[6] The number of specialist voluntary sector and acute trust-based providers varies widely between PCTs, as do the number of host organisations of specialist palliative home care teams, which include PCTs themselves, neighbouring PCTs, acute trusts and voluntary hospices. Such organisational complexity has implications for the commissioning of palliative care by PCTs. It can also limit healthcare professionals' awareness of services, and have an impact on effective communication and joint working between providers (see Figures 10.1 and 10.2).

Since the 1995 Calman–Hine report, the organisation and delivery of cancer services has also been subject to rapid change.[3,7] Cancer Networks were established to give a strategic overview of the commissioning and provision of cancer services, serving populations of around one and a half million in implementing the recommendations of the NHS Cancer Plan. Cancer Networks bring together PCT commissioners with providers to develop service delivery plans across all aspects of cancer care, including palliative care. Separate palliative care sub-committees are therefore placed within the Cancer Network structure, despite the government's acknowledgement of the palliative care needs of non-cancer patients.[5]

### The commissioning cycle

Commissioning is the process through which PCTs 'identify the health needs of their population and make prioritised decisions to secure care to meet those needs within available resources'.[8] It involves two major activities – the planning of services, and the

Figure 10.1 **Palliative care system one: example of a system with few providers[6]**

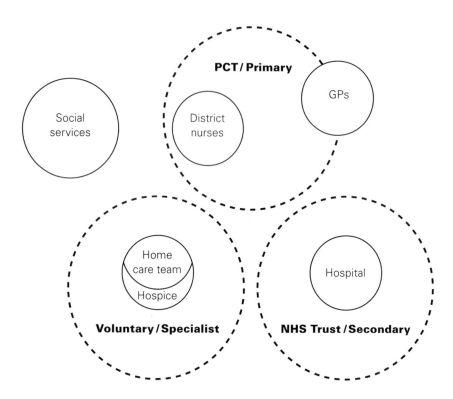

Services involved in providing palliative care in this area:

**primary care sector**
- GPs semi-autonomous but contracted to PCT
- district nurses employed by PCT

**NHS trust/secondary sector**
- one hospital palliative care team serving PCT

**voluntary/specialist sector**
- one in-patient hospice with home care team serving PCT

Figure 10.2 **Palliative care system two: example of a system with multiple providers[6]**

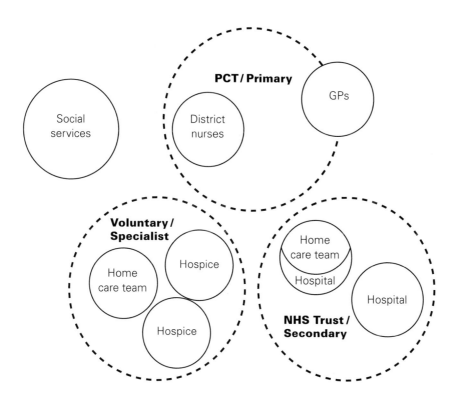

**primary care sector**
- GPs semi-autonomous but contracted to PCT
- district nurses employed by PCT

**NHS trust/secondary sector**
- two hospital palliative care teams serving PCT – one with home care team attached

**voluntary/specialist sector**
- three in-patient hospices serving PCT – one with home care team attached

Figure 10.3 **The commissioning cycle**

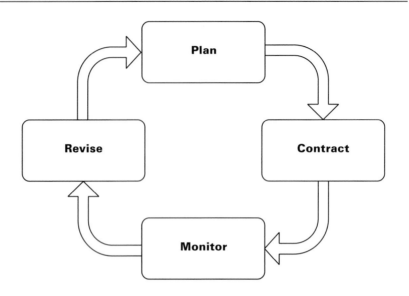

contracting of services. PCTs work within what is commonly referred to as the 'commissioning cycle' in order to achieve these.

Of the four phases of the commissioning cycle, *planning* is perhaps the most complex and time consuming. Planners must address a number of different key questions, including:

- health needs assessment – do current resources meet identified needs?
- health equity audit – are resources and services distributed equitably, in relation to health needs of different groups and areas?
- national targets – what needs to be done to meet key national targets?
- current provision – how are services currently provided?
- capacity planning – how might demand change and what impact would this have?
- comparative performance – do services represent value for money?

These strands are brought together into a Local Delivery Plan (LDP), a three-year plan of service delivery for the PCT that forms the basis of future commissioning decisions.

The next stage of the commissioning cycle – contracting – requires PCTs to draw up Service Level Agreements (SLAs) with all providers, negotiated in relation to the Local Delivery Plan (volumes, quality and cost of care). These SLAs are then monitored, and revised in light of reported activity. Running throughout this cycle is the importance of consulting with local populations in the planning and contracting of all services.[8]

The commissioning cycle may take place for certain healthcare services at the level of the individual PCT. However, the complexity and volume of many healthcare service areas requires PCTs to join together to commission services. This may be done in one of four ways:

1. joint or collaborative commissioning, where PCTs devise a framework within which they commission particular services jointly

2. lead commissioning, with one organisation acting as 'lead' on behalf of a group of PCTs

3. consortia commissioning, where another organisational body is created and funded by a group of organisations to commission on their behalf

4. shared services, where a new, separate organisation is created to commission on behalf of PCTs.

The decision as to which is the best way to commission particular services will depend on the nature of that service. For example, out-of-hours care – with a wide range of providers, most of whom work across PCT boundaries – can be commissioned collaboratively by groups of PCTs, especially in inner-city areas such as London. Palliative care needs assessments and service planning will be taken forward at the level of Cancer Networks, although in practice these Network plans may be difficult to implement locally due to resource restraints, both financial and human. Many PCTs will contract individually with providers to supply services for their populations.

---

Box 10.1 **Payment by Results – an overview**

---

Payment by Results will require a major change of approach to commissioning services. PCTs will commission the precise volume of clinical activity they require, from a number of different providers. PCTs will pay a standard 'national tariff', adjusted for case mix, and this funding will flow to providers based on the actual care they deliver. The scheme is rolling out from elective in-patient care, through non-elective in-patient, out-patient, A&E and ambulance, and community care, becoming fully operational by 2008/9.

The key principles of payment by results are:

**1** a standard national tariff, with prices adjusted for:

- cost pressures (as the base data from which the tariff is derived will always be up to two years in arrears)

- long stay outliers, or exceptional cases

- critical care costs

- specialist work

**2** tariff prices to reflect case mix, based on Healthcare Resource Groups (HRGs)

**3** cost and volume commissioning, specifying the amount of activity (based on HRGs) and the price the PCT will pay (based on the standard national tariff).

---

*Source*: adapted from the Audit Commission. *Getting the Balance Right for the NHS and Taxpayers*. Introducing payment by results. London: Audit Commission, 2004.

## The new commissioning environment

Whilst the section above outlines the basic approach to commissioning services, the commissioning *environment* within which PCTs must plan and secure services is changing. The gradual introduction of standard national tariffs for most service activity, known as 'Payment by Results', from 2003 onwards requires the negotiation of radically different SLAs between PCTs and providers (see Box 10.1).[9] National price tariffs set by the Department of Health use Health-care Resource Group (HRG) classifications to group care received by patients, and services are commissioned by PCTs on a case mix – weighted cost and volume basis. All providers will therefore be reimbursed according to the numbers of patients they treat; in effect, the 'money' follows the 'patient' as opposed to block amounts being given to providers. As a result, Payment by Results requires both PCTs and providers to manage the risk. PCTs will have the difficult task of managing demand and overperformance, and the financial consequences, whereas providers will have to manage the risks associated with underactivity, which may not allow for the tariff to cover full costs of a service.

Within the acute care sector, Payment by Results is strongly linked to the Patient Choice agenda. From 2005, patients referred for planned hospital care have been able to choose from between four to five alternate providers, at the point of booking their appointment.[10] The impact of patient choice in reimbursing providers and financial flows could be substantial, with PCTs required to produce much more detailed estimates of demand to assist their planning. However, the government's prioritisation of patient choice is not limited to offering options about the place of care in the acute sector; it also includes the private sector. The importance placed on giving patients the choice to be cared for and die at home if they so wish, as outlined in the government's End-of-Life Programme, also places a responsibility on PCTs to commission services in order to meet these aims.[11] These initiatives are all aimed at improving the access and quality of services to patients.

The introduction of Practice-Based Commissioning, another key health service reform, has added further complexity to the commissioning cycle.[12] From April 2005, GP practices could, on request, receive an indicative budget from their PCT.[13] The aim is for all practices to be involved in Practice-Based Commissioning by 2008, with budgets used to 'directly manage the delivery of services for their patients'.[14] Whilst PCTs hold the actual budget, and continue to negotiate service-level agreements, practices may ultimately make commissioning decisions over the entire scope of healthcare provision, with the exception of a few highly specialised services. Practices may choose to hold their own budget and make all decisions, or join with other practices in a locality to commission services between them. As Smith *et al.* note, these arrangements may lead PCTs in future to act simply as a receiving house, dividing out the NHS budget between sub-commissioning groups including practices or localities, and macro-commissioning arrangements for more specialist services.[15]

That is, PCTs could effectively become the 'contracting' department.

Practice-based locality or cluster commissioning plans (PBC) must be developed alongside PCT LDPs. Although not explicitly dictated by the LDP, PBC commissioning plans must support and complement the LDP, and they must be signed off by the PCT board. It is also important to ensure that the local healthcare infrastructure is not disadvantaged by PBC, and that one locality/cluster does not suffer adverse consequences by the commissioning 'desires' of another. As a result, there will need to be an open and transparent process of a competitive market for the provision of services. A PBC cluster will not automatically be able to provide a service within their locality, but will need to bid alongside other providers, necessitating evidence of a quality, cost-effective service to the whole health economy. Furthermore, the PBC localities/clusters will be responsible for ensuring national targets are reached; these must be taken into account when formulating their commissioning plans.

**Commissioning unscheduled care: key 'must-do's'**

A further major commissioning challenge for PCTs in recent years has been the development of integrated systems of unscheduled and emergency care services, in line with the Reforming Emergency Care Strategy and the Carson report on GP out-of-hours services.[16,17] Such systems encompass both in- and out-of-hours services, and include:

- the provision of immediate access care, particularly primary care, in hours
- the provision of immediate access care, particularly primary care, out of hours
- the provision of A & E services
- the development of admission avoidance policies

The aim of all such systems is to enable any individual requiring unplanned, urgent medical care to be directed towards 'the right person, with the right skills, in the right place, at the right time, preferably at the time of first contact'.[16]

The need for PCTs to ensure the provision of coordinated, appropriate care was intensified following the introduction of the new General Medical Services contract in April 2004.[18] This enabled all

GP practices to opt out of providing 24-hour care for their patients, with PCTs taking over this responsibility. In taking on this new role, PCTs were encouraged to commission out-of-hours service providers employing a greater skill mix than the previous GP-led services.

In any one urgent care system a multitude of providers are involved in offering treatment and support to patients with need for immediate care. These providers include:

- GP practices
- accredited out-of-hours primary care service providers
- A & E departments
- ambulance services
- district nursing services
- NHS Direct
- specialist palliative care services
- social services
- mental health services
- minor injury units
- walk-in centres
- pharmacists
- dental services
- intermediate care services
- rapid response and hospital at home services.

Many of these providers will cover more than one PCT. Collaborative commissioning arrangements, with PCTs working together with others to secure services, are therefore necessary to engage with all providers and deliver integrated services. Such partnerships have often developed under the auspices of Urgent and Emergency Care Networks (ECNs), bringing together providers and commissioners in the same way as Cancer Networks.

### In-hours unscheduled care

Under the NHS Plan targets, from 2004 all patients should be able to see a primary care professional within 24 hours of requesting an appointment, and a GP within 48 hours.[2] A model of care designed to enable this – the *Advanced Access* model developed by the National

Primary Care Development Team – aims to assist practices in identifying the pattern of demand for their services, and work to match their capacity to this.[19] The goal is to offer a same-day appointment to all patients, regardless of whether their need is 'urgent' or 'routine'. Perhaps in deference to concerns about continuity of care, the NHS Plan targets also allow patients to wait longer than 48 hours to see a GP of their choice, if necessary. However, the major impact of the access targets is to shift the emphasis away from 'own-GP' care to the receipt of timely care from any member of the primary healthcare team. This shift is further compounded by the new GMS contract, with patients now registered with a practice rather than an individual GP.[18] In negotiating contracts with each GMS practice, PCTs will need to ensure that they are able to attain the essential primary medical services that form the core of the new contract, including the general management of patients who are terminally ill, although quite what this comprises is less than clear. It will be particularly important for practices to ensure that, in meeting access targets, they also meet the requirements of their patients with palliative care needs – again, this will be difficult to measure. This may be an opportune time for practices to implement a framework – for example, the Gold Standards Framework (see Chapter 11) – within their practice, and to ensure that palliative care needs are included in their commissioning plans. Incentives for practices to do so now exist through additional Quality and Outcomes Framework points for palliative care.

### Out-of-hours unscheduled care

As a result of the new GP contract and the Reforming Emergency Care agenda, PCTs must offer an integrated system of unscheduled and emergency care, from 18.30 to 08.00 on weekdays, and all day at the weekends and bank holidays, to meet the needs of their local population. This system will include an accredited out-of-hours provider or providers to offer first-point-of-contact primary care to patients with a need for urgent treatment or advice. Accredited providers may emerge from the previous GP cooperatives or deputising services, although in line with policy guidance they will employ much greater skill mix than previous services. In response to this requirement, and the resulting innovations in providing care, out-of-hours services have become more diverse across areas. This diversification of services has in part been driven by differential responses to local needs and the availability and use of staff. Options being explored may include emergency care practitioners taking over some aspects of GP care, an enhanced role for district nurses, and the use of specialist nurses in home visits – such as for patients with palliative care needs. All services, however, must meet the quality standards for out-of-hours care set out by the Department of Health.[20] PCTs need to liaise with other health and social care providers including A & E, ambulance and specialist palliative care services to ensure a seamless service meets the needs of all patients. As the Carson review of GP out-of-hours services envisaged, systems should enable single-call access to out-of-hours care (excluding 999 calls), either through NHS Direct or another provider. Strategic Health Authorities were tasked with performance managing new arrangements for out-of-hours care, ensuring that PCTs collaborate effectively within the context of the ECN.

Coordination of services and sharing of information are vital to the success of these systems. The sharing of information is crucial to ensure continuity of care for patients, particularly vulnerable patient groups such as those with palliative care needs. One of the quality standards is that providers must implement systems to exchange up-to-date and comprehensive information on patients with predefined needs, including those with terminal illness.[20]

## Commissioning palliative care: current and future challenges

Specialist palliative care services are currently planned at the level of the Cancer Network, in consultation with PCTs, Strategic Health Authorities and providers; effective palliative care planning and funding can be dependent on larger populations than those covered by individual PCTs. Current planning procedures follow the Department of Health's requirements for the distribution of an extra £50 million per annum investment in specialist palliative care from 2003/4.[21] The original three-year plans, running from 2003/4 to 2005/6, had to take into account the draft NICE guidance on supportive and palliative care – published in full in March 2004.[5] More recently, guidance on needs assessment for specialist palliative care services has been published by the National Hospice Council to help Networks decide on their level of population need for these services, and the likely capacity required to meet these needs, in order to inform future commissioning and the implementation of the NICE guidance.[22]

Key recommendations contained within the NICE guidance highlight the complexity of the challenge faced by PCTs and Networks in fulfilling their commissioning role in palliative care. For example:

Key recommendation 3:

Each multidisciplinary team or service should implement processes to ensure effective inter-professional communication within teams and between them and other service providers with whom the patient has contact. Mechanisms should be developed to promote continuity of care, which might include the nomination of a person to take on the role of 'key worker' for individual patients.

Key Recommendation 12:

Mechanisms need to be implemented within each locality to ensure that medical and nursing services are available for patients with advanced cancer on a 24-hour, seven days a week basis, and that equipment can be provided without undue delay. Those providing generalist medical and nursing services should have access to specialist advice at all times.[5]

The recommendations above focus on the importance of good communication between services, and the need to provide both generalist and specialist palliative care. However, generalist palliative care is not a distinct service that can be assessed and defined by commissioners. It is part of the everyday practice of healthcare professionals, such as district and community nurses and GPs, and cannot therefore be planned and contracted in the same way as specialist palliative care. Yet it is fundamental to caring for the majority of patients with palliative care needs, who will spend most of their final year of life at home under the care of the primary healthcare team.[23] Recognising the importance of palliative care for professionals such as district nurses is essential if PCTs are to ensure adequate capacity in these services. This is especially pertinent to the current drive to provide the opportunity for patients to die at home if they so wish.[11]

However, the situation is further complicated as, whilst care of dying patients is viewed as a rewarding and important part of the work of GPs, it makes up a small proportion of their overall workload.[24,25] Additionally, GPs may choose varying ways of working with specialist palliative care services, for example:

a)  using specialist services only infrequently

b)  using specialist services as a resource (the most common model)

c)  working with specialist services as an extended team

d)  handing over care or responsibility to specialist services.[26]

These models of care are shaped by the current context within which the GP is working, and GPs may therefore employ alternative approaches at varying times.

A recent King's Fund report into the provision of palliative care within primary care found that relationships between generalist and specialist providers could at times be poor, with breakdowns in communication and misunderstandings of roles.[6] It stressed the important function of PCTs in clarifying roles and responsibilities between providers, in developing standards of care, and in thinking creatively about the use of innovations such as GPs with Special Interests, the commissioning of locally enhanced services, or an increased role for specialist services to meet the palliative care needs of their populations.

An additional consideration for PCTs is the increasing interest in the palliative care needs of non-cancer patients.[23,27] The mechanisms for commissioning palliative care are situated within the service planning and delivery structures set up to deliver the key targets of the NHS Cancer Plan. Around 95 per cent of specialist palliative in-patient and home care patients have a diagnosis of cancer.[28] The NICE guidance is aimed at cancer patients, although many of its requirements will benefit non-cancer patients as well. Including the needs of non-cancer patients in the commissioning of palliative care services remains challenging. However, in a number of National

Service Frameworks (NSFs), such as the Coronary Heart Disease NSF and the Long Term Conditions NSF, there is a requirement to ensure palliative care provision.

The Department of Health is planning to implement Payment by Results for adult palliative care, across both the NHS and voluntary sector, by 2008/9. Funding will therefore follow patient numbers and be influenced, potentially, by patients' choices both of special-ist palliative care provider, and of location of care (such as in the community). Within the acute sector, Payment by Results is designed to make the patient choice agenda 'bite' on providers – with poorer services losing funding as patients choose to go elsewhere. There is a risk that similar, formal competition will also be introduced to pal-liative care – especially in areas with a number of specialist palliative care services.

The impact of these changes on the creation of systems aiming to foster continuity of care for palliative care patients is, by necessity, speculative. One area where positive developments may occur is in the flow of information: Payment by Results will require high-quality data on clinical activity, and thus the further development of existing information systems. However, potential adverse outcomes include threats to the quality and flexibility of care provided, as setting the national tariff too low could force providers to make cuts in level of service to stay within budget. Furthermore, the effect of funding 100 per cent of the national tariff for NHS palliative care services, and a possible 50 per cent of the tariff to voluntary sector services, on the type and level of care available to patients under these two options remains unexplored. A more competitive environment could strain collaborative relationships between services. It also remains to be seen how well palliative care activity can be measured, and how well integrated care functions within a Payment by Results system when episodes of care are bought.

However, Practice-Based Commissioning may offer a positive mechanism to improve continuity of care. With the decision making resting with GPs, guided by detailed knowledge of the experiences of their palliative care patients, new approaches to providing cohe-sive palliative care services could be fostered. Innovations could include the provision of a specific primary palliative care service, commissioned by GPs in one locality in conjunction with local specialist providers, providing care both in and out of hours. GPs could even employ their own clinical nurse specialist. However, any new palliative care service developments would necessitate GP localities first making savings through reduced referrals to secondary care, before they were free to spend money on new initiatives. Furthermore, they would not automatically be able to take over these roles, as there would need to be an open and transparent tendering process agreed by PCT Boards. This may restrict their ability to implement major changes at will.

### Meeting the challenge

Achievement of an integrated system that meets the needs of all patients under the 'right person, right skills, right place' model, including high-quality specialist palliative care round the clock, is dependent on effective commissioning of services by PCTs in the first instance, and subsequently to be followed through Practice-Based Commissioning. In 2004, the Health Select Committee queried the readiness and commitment of PCTs to take on the responsibility of commissioning out-of-hours services.[29] The Audit Commission has also questioned both the management capacity of PCTs, and the adequacy of financial planning undertaken by them.[30,31] This reflects more global concerns about the performance of PCTs in carrying out their major functions.[32] In part, questions about the effectiveness of PCTs in commissioning services arise from the numerous reorganisations that have been imposed on commissioning bodies in recent years, whilst providers have remained relatively stable.[15] Without core stability, it can be difficult to have sufficient organisational maturity and adequate expertise to tackle commissioning, and in particular the planning of services, effectively.[15] There is a constant moving of 'goal posts', occurring to an even greater extent from 2006. This creates a very insecure foundation for implementing the forthcoming developments, and ensuring continuity and quality of patient care.

As this chapter was being written, the Department of Health has suggested in *Commissioning a Patient-Led NHS* that PCTs may lose some or all of their provider functions.[33] Should all provider functions be reorganised, this may well have profound implications for the structure of primary and community palliative care. This would affect the provision of district nursing services, central to supporting patients at home, and in some instances the provision of specialist palliative care. In responding to anxieties generated by the announcement, four months later the Department of Health apologised for being too prescriptive and said that such decision making will be left to PCTs.[34] The outcome of these negotiations is very unclear – although it could lead to a radical reorganisation of community care, with greater involvement of the independent and voluntary sector, and threats to continuity of care as a result of the fracturing of important links between services.

Within this context of organisational immaturity and instability, a review of the targets PCTs are required to meet provides further insight into the time and attention PCTs are able to direct towards palliative care. Under the Department of Health's Priorities and Planning Framework 2003–6, issued in 2002, PCTs – along with other NHS and social care organisations – were required to plan for the delivery of 44 key targets covering improving access, cancer, coronary heart disease, mental health, older people, life chances for children, improving patient experience, regional health inequalities, and drugs misuse.[35] PCT progress is checked and rated by the Healthcare Commission – in 2005, these ratings were based on eight key targets and a further 33 'balanced scorecard' indicators of PCT performance. Palliative care, whilst it has received attention in recent years as a result of the NICE guidance and the Building on the Best Initiative,[5,11] has only featured from 2006 in such major drivers of PCT commitment and work.

## Conclusions and ways forward

In commissioning all healthcare services, PCTs and Networks are encouraged to think through the 'patient pathway' to understand the service elements or 'touch points' that need to come together to provide care.[8] An integrated approach is particularly crucial in areas with a diverse array of service providers and settings, such as palliative care. The possibilities for an interruption in continuity of care are inevitably more numerous where patients require care from primary, secondary and voluntary sector providers, on a both scheduled and

unscheduled basis. The impact of forthcoming plans to both restruc-
ture some PCTs and reduce provider functions is as yet unknown.

Whilst the NICE guidance has provided impetus to develop higher
standards of more integrated care, the major change in financing of
services due to Payment by Results may have a destabilising effect
in future. Partnership working is crucial if PCTs are to meet the
challenge of commissioning both palliative care and out-of-hours
services. This is necessary both between providers and PCTs, at the
level of primary health care and palliative care teams, and between
individuals. The expertise of Cancer Networks in the subject of palliative care is also critical in supporting PCT commissioners who
may lack sufficient expertise in this area. Additionally, specialist palliative care providers will be important sources of energy, knowledge
and commitment in ensuring the needs of palliative care patients are
met; yet all this needs to be done in an environment where shortage
of skilled staff in palliative care is at its highest. All these initiatives
are aimed at improving access to and quality of services for patients,
and commissioners and providers will have to keep this goal firmly
in mind as they navigate through the ever-changing environment in
which they work.

## Summary

- PCTs are key organisations in the planning and commissioning
  of palliative care services – yet palliative care forms a very small
  part of their total responsibilities.

- Effective commissioning of services is integral to ensuring effective continuity of palliative care.

- However, the commissioning environment in which PCTs plan
  and contract services is changing rapidly.

- In particular, the introduction of initiatives such as Payment by
  Results, Practice-Based Commissioning, the development of integrated systems of unscheduled and emergency care, and further
  changes to the organisational structure of PCTs, are all potential
  opportunities for, or threats to, the continuity of primary palliative care.

**REFERENCES**

1. DoH. *Shifting the Balance of Power: Securing delivery*. London: Department of Health, 2001.

2. DoH. *The NHS Plan. A plan for investment. A plan for reform*. London: Department of Health, 2000.

3. DoH. *The NHS Cancer Plan. A plan for investment. A plan for reform*. London: Department of Health, 2000.

4. DoH. *National Service Framework for Older People*. London: Department of Health, 2001, pp. 1–202.

5. NICE. *Guidance on Cancer Services. Improving supportive and palliative care for adults with cancer*. London: National Institute for Clinical Excellence, 2004.

6. Burt J, Shipman C, Addington-Hall J and White P. *Palliative Care: Perspectives on caring for dying people in London*. London: King's Fund, 2005.

7. Calman K and Hine D. *A Policy Framework for Commissioning Cancer Services*. London: Department of Health, 1995.

8. NATPACT. *The Commissioning Friend for PCTs. Whole system commissioning of acute services*. London: National Primary and Care Trust Development Programme, 2004.

9. DoH. *Reforming NHS Financial Flows. Introducing Payment by Results*. London: Department of Health, 2002.

10. DoH. *'Choose and Book' – Patient's choice of hospital and booked appointment. Policy framework for choice and booking at the point of referral*. London: Department of Health, 2004.

11. DoH. *Building on the Best: End of Life Care Initiative*. London: Department of Health, 2004.

12. DoH. *Practice Based Commissioning. Promoting clinical engagement*. London: Department of Health, 2004.

13. DoH. *The NHS Improvement Plan. Putting people at the heart of public services*. London: The Stationery Office, 2004.

14. DoH. *Making Practice Based Commissioning a Reality. Technical guidance*. London: Department of Health, 2005.

15. Smith J, Mays N, Dixon J, Goodwin N, Lewis R, McClelland S, *et al. A Review of the Effectiveness of Primary Care-Led Commissioning and Its Place in the NHS*. London: The Health Foundation, 2004, pp. 1–57.

16. DoH. *Reforming Emergency Care. First steps to a new approach*. London: Department of Health, 2001.

17. DoH. *Raising Standards for Patients. New partnerships in out-of-hours care. An independent review of GP out-of-hours services in England*. London: Department of Health, 2000.

18.  DoH. *Investing in General Practice. The new General Medical Services contract*. London: Department of Health, 2003.

19.  Oldham J. *Advanced Access in Primary Care*. Manchester: Advanced Access in Primary Care, 2001.

20.  DoH. *National Quality Requirements in the Delivery of Out-of-Hours Services*. London: Department of Health, 2004.

21.  DoH. *Planning and Funding Specialist Palliative Care Provision 2003/04–2005/06*. London: Department of Health, 2004.

22.  Tebbit P. *Population-Based Needs Assessment for Palliative Care – A manual for Cancer Networks*. London: The National Council for Palliative Care and the Cancer Action Team, 2004.

23.  Barclay S. Palliative care for non-cancer patients: A UK perspective from primary care. In: Addington-Hall J and Higginson I, eds. *Palliative Care for Non-Cancer Patients*. Oxford: Oxford University Press, 2001, pp. 172–88.

24.  Field D and McGaughey J. An evaluation of palliative care services for cancer patients in the Southern Health and Social Services Board of Northern Ireland. *Palliative Medicine* 1998; **12 (2)**: 83–97.

25.  Lloyd-Williams M. General Practitioners in North Wales: Current experiences of palliative care. *European Journal of Cancer Care* 2000; **9**: 138–43.

26.  Shipman C, Addington-Hall J, Barclay S, Briggs J, Daniels L and Millar D. How and why do GPs use specialist palliative care services? *Palliative Medicine* 2002; **16 (3)**: 241–6.

27.  Addington-Hall J, Fakhoury W and McCarthy M. Specialist palliative care in nonmalignant disease. *Palliative Medicine* 1998; **12 (6)**: 417–27.

28.  Care TNCfP. *National Survey of Patient Activity Data for Specialist Palliative Care Services. Full report for the year 2003–2004*. London: The National Council for Palliative Care, 2005.

29.  Committee HoCH. *GP Out-of-Hours Services. Fifth report of session 2003–04*. London: The Stationery Office, 2004.

30.  Commission A. *Achieving the NHS Plan: Assessment of current performance, likely future progress and capacity to improve*. London: Audit Commission, 2003.

31.  Commission A. *Financial Management in the NHS*. London: Audit Commission, 2004.

32.  Roche D. *PCTs: An unfinished agenda*. London: Institute for Public Policy Research, 2004.

33.  Department of Health. *Commissioning a Patient-Led NHS*. London: Department of Health, 28 July 2005.

34.  *Health Service Journal*, 17 November 2005, p. 7.

35.  DoH. *Improvement, Expansion and Reform: The next three years' priorities and planning framework, 2003–2006*. London: Department of Health, 2002.

CHAPTER | 11

# End-of-life initiatives and continuity in primary palliative care

*Kashifa Mahmood and Dan Munday*

## Introduction

Patients with advanced cancer and other chronic illnesses that have reached a terminal stage have high levels of healthcare need. Many may have repeated and sometimes prolonged admission to hospital or hospices, but the majority will spend at least 90 per cent of their last year of life in their own homes,[1] receiving medical and nursing care from primary and community specialist teams. General practitioners[2,3] and district nurses (DNs)[4-6] have seen care of dying patients as an integral part of their role. The service they offer the dying patient is part of a generalist approach to health care and is provided in the midst of attending to other patients with a wide variety of conditions: acute and chronic, minor and serious, physical and psychological, in the context of family and social relationships. In addition GPs and community nurses will have a role in preventative health and surveillance, and will be concerned with the whole practice population in addition to the individual patient. The modern GP has been described by McWhinney as 'a new kind of hybrid practitioner with competencies in primary care, prevention, epidemiology, ethics and behavioural science'.[7]

GPs may care for four or five terminally ill cancer patients each year and will have 10 to 20 patients who die with chronic non-cancer illness. Increasingly specialist treatment has become available for many potentially life-threatening conditions, including oncological treatments for cancer. In addition, specialist teams in the community have provided alternatives to primary care, such that GPs in particular may become less involved with terminally ill patients than they were formerly, which has threatened their role as personal physician to their patients. The risk to patients of accessing services offered by many different professionals and teams is that care may become fragmented despite good coordination of services.

The recent changes to the GP contract are potentially changing the nature of general practice dramatically.[8] Some commentators are concerned that the new contract fails to give palliative care sufficient priority[9] and others that it is potentially threatening continuity of care.[10] Payment through the Quality and Outcomes Framework (QOF) may encourage GPs to concentrate on achieving defined process and outcome measures in screening, health promotion and chronic disease management, putting holistic care, which is less easily measured, at risk.[11]

Other recent drives to improve quality in health care have focused on defining best practice based on a systematic synthesis of research evidence, particularly through initiatives such as the Cochrane Collaboration and National Institute for Health and Clinical Excellence (NICE). Quality is increasingly defined in the National Service Frameworks (NSF) for the management of specific conditions and patient groups.[12] These have included guidance for the management of patients in the palliative stages of their illnesses.[3,4,13] Whilst guidelines and frameworks have highlighted the importance of continuity of care and a multidisciplinary teamwork approach in palliative care, few have addressed the issue of how these aspects are maintained.

This chapter will examine recent initiatives, the Gold Standards Framework for Palliative Care (GSF), Preferred Place of Care Tool (PPOC) and Liverpool Care of the Dying Pathway (LCP), focusing on aspects of these programmes that aim to improve continuity of care. These programmes are designed to empower generalist practitioners to improve care for patients with advanced disease and terminal illness, and have been adopted by the NHS End-of-Life Care Programme (EoLCP), which is also described in this chapter. Particular focus will be paid to the GSF, which is a major development in primary palliative care.

In view of the centrality of patient choice within these frameworks and since determinants of place of death have been the subject of a number of research studies in the last 15 years, the next section will briefly explore some of the insights and issues that have emerged.

## Preferred place of death

Studies have suggested that whilst many patients would prefer to die at home only 25 per cent actually do so.[14-16] Many complex issues have been shown to underlie this statistic and research has concentrated on developing insights into which patients are more likely to achieve a home death and which are not.[16-18]

Fulfilling place of death preferences requires the availability of an array of services that have to be effectively coordinated in order to empower choice and provide opportunities for patients to express their wishes. The logistical factors to be considered in promoting the quality of care as well as choice for patients with end-stage disease is outlined in several studies. Higginson and Sen-Gupta[19] reviewed the literature on preferred place of care for the terminally ill, yielding evidence from studies of variable quality with diverse approaches. The majority of studies of the highest quality suggested the preference for home death rate was between 50–90 per cent. The studies reviewed highlighted the problematic nature of conceptualising and measuring fulfilment of place of death preferences. The authors suggest that a preference for home care may be an empowered expression of wishes, or may reflect an aversion to the perceived disadvantages of hospital care. Choice of dying in a hospital or hospice may indicate a desire to relieve the family in their caring role. In certain studies involving terminally ill patients, a preference for home death decreased and an acceptance of an in-patient death increased over time.[20] Preferences may be tempered by changes in patient circumstances as the disease progressed. The preference for *home care* appeared to be higher than for death at home and these options were strongly influenced by the services provided. Organisational factors may therefore combine with patient choice to affect home death rates. Statistics need to be interpreted with caution as the quality of care needs to be evaluated in whichever setting patients choose to die.

Empirical data drawn from the narrative accounts of the parents of 13 young adult patients who died of cancer illustrated that informal support, capacity to care and expression of strong preferences make a home death more probable in the young adult age group.[21] The findings reinforced an analysis of 10-year trends in the place of death of cancer patients which revealed that older people and women were less likely to die at home than younger adults and men.[16] Karlsen and

Addington-Hall[18] noted in a post-bereavement survey conducted of 229 people using the VOICES (Views of Informal Carers – Evaluation of Services) questionnaire that patients requiring health and social service support with self-care tasks (a proxy for high levels of frailty and dependency) were less likely to achieve a home death. It was concluded that support at home produced the strongest influence on place of death, with nursing and social service provision in the home being the most significant aspect.

A potential weakness of studies into preferred place of death is the lack of clarity on how patient preferences are elicited and therefore recorded.[19] Thomas et al.,[22] in a study of the preferences of 41 terminally ill cancer patients and 18 of their informal carers in Northwest England, highlighted the complexities surrounding the concept of preferred place of death. Familiar themes emerged indicating that patient choices were influenced by contextual factors including: the extent of the patient's social network; perception of carer's attitude; symptom management; fear of loss of dignity; and view of hospices, nursing homes, hospitals and the reliability of community services. However, patient choices were also characterised by uncertainty and 'preferences were rarely stated categorically, but took the form of a stronger or weaker leaning in one direction' qualified by speculation as to how this may change with events. They therefore challenged the view that preferences could be considered in the abstract, with patients 'taking a pragmatic view, acknowledging the contingency at work in their lives'.[22] Patient preferences were shaped by constraints even before choices were articulated to professionals. An additional paper by Thomas[23] reported the results of semi-structured interviews with 15 palliative care providers in Morecambe Bay that illuminated how the values, behaviour and information provided by referring practitioners could steer patients into particular care settings and influence preferred place of death. Providers identify and weigh alternative criteria in order to reach the optimal decision.[24]

Determining preferred place of death does not appear to be a simple process since it seems to be contingent on many factors and is likely to change over time. Open communication enabling careful exploration of important issues for the individual patient and constant review of patient preferences all require awareness and skill on the part of the attending health professional. Little appears to be

known of how professionals deal with the issues that arise from elic-
iting a patient's preferred place of death. More research is required in
this area if the aspirations of enabling patients to choose where they
die is to be realised.

### The NHS End-of-Life Care Programme (EoLCP)

In December 2003 the UK Department of Health published a paper
*Building on the Best: Choice, responsiveness and equity in the NHS* out-
lining how the government aimed to make NHS services more
responsive to patients by providing more choice across the spectrum
of health care, from birth to death. The explicit aim for end-of-life
care was 'to offer all adult patients nearing the end of life, regardless
of their diagnosis, the same access to high quality palliative care *so
that they can choose if they wish to die at home'.*[25]
   The same month the Secretary of State for Health announced an
initiative for which a £12 million investment over three years to
improve the care of people in the final stages of their lives was to be
made. This led to the establishment of the EoLCP in November 2004,
the aims of which are to:

- expand choice for patients in terms of where they want to live
  and die irrespective of their diagnosis
- decrease the number of emergency admissions of patients who
  expressly wish to die at home
- reduce the number of older people transferred from a care
  home to a district general hospital in the last week of life.

   The three frameworks endorsed by NICE Guidance for Supportive and Palliative Care were identified for implementation by the
EoLCP: GSF, PPOC and LCP. The GSF has also been accredited by
the Royal College of General Practitioners (RCGP).

   Through the EoLCP these frameworks are being implemented
within both community and institutional settings, with the investment designated to facilitate this process.

### Preferred Place of Care Tool (PPOC)

The PPOC was designed by Lancashire and South Cumbria Cancer Network and arises out of a programme of DN training to raise the quality of palliative care. The primary aim of the tool is to allow professionals, patients and carers to plan a total package of care (see Box 11.1).[26] The PPOC tool is designed as a patient-held record that remains with patients through the trajectory of their care. The document enables patients to be at the centre of the plan, thereby engendering autonomy and control for them and carers. It enables services to be focused on patients' preferences and for the outcomes to be audited.[27] Discussion of the issues in the document with the DN allows an evolving plan to develop as the situation changes. It strives to strengthen continuity of service through the provision of information to out-of-hours services. The tool also provides 'qualitative' data to identify whether or not patients died at their preferred location. The developers acknowledge the difficulty of demonstrating a causal link between the results of the initiative and changes in patient outcomes and experiences due to the complex nature of the situations encountered. The plan is to audit the number of patients

---

Box 11.1 **Preferred Place of Care Tool**

- The document collates the demographic data relating to the patient. It requests gender, postcode, date of birth and GP, and maintains the anonymity of the patient during data analysis by the Cancer Network project team. A family profile section explores circumstances relating to dependants and identifies the key carer(s).

- The second section facilitates discussion with the patient and family on their understanding of the diagnosis and possible outcomes. The practitioner explores patient and family preferences regarding the setting in which to be cared for and by whom when the patient's condition starts to deteriorate. This process will evolve over time but may never be fully addressed for patients in denial.

- The third section facilitates a comprehensive assessment of health and social services available to the patient, and identifies which if any are currently being accessed.

- Finally, a variance sheet allows the patient and professional to document changes in the need for services. Comments are invited about the services.

---

*Source*: Storey et al.,[26] p. 38.    Reproduced by kind permission of the RCN Publishing Company.

dying at home, in hospital or hospice in the five years preceding and following the implementation of the initiative.

## Liverpool Care Pathway

The LCP is a method of delivering holistic care during the dying phase of a terminal illness. It gives guidance for staff on various aspects of care (see Box 11.2), provides a framework for reviewing clinical progression and through its documentation helps to ensure continuity between professionals involved in delivering care. When a patient is placed on the LCP other methods of documentation such as doctor's case notes and nurse's care plans are replaced, and team members are expecte to write in the care pathway instead. The documentation is available for auditing the process and outcomes of care thereby offering a tool for continued learning.

It is suggested that patients should be placed on the LCP when signs of dying are apparent. These include: the patient becomes bed-bound, semi-comatose and only able to take sips of fluid and cannot swallow tablets. The prescription of 'as required' medication is advised for pain, nausea/vomiting and respiratory tract secretions. In addition, medication of the dying patient should be reviewed and non-essential drugs discontinued. Patients should be reviewed at least every four hours to ensure that they have good symptom control, with action taken if this has not been achieved.

Finally, the care pathway highlights the need to clearly communicate with the family that the patient is dying and provide support and information through the terminal phase, and when the patient has died. Kinder and Ellershaw[28] outlined the key points for reviewing palliative patients according to the LCP found in Box 11.2.

The LCP, whilst initially designed to be used in the in-patient setting, particularly as a tool for generalist staff to enable them to provide high-quality palliative care, has been successfully adapted and used in many settings, including the community and within care homes.[29] It has also been adopted as an integral component of the GSF for Palliative Care.

---

Box 11.2 **LCP – Initial assessment and care goals**

---

**Comfort measures**

Goal 1: current medication assessed and non-essentials discontinued.

Goal 2: 'as required' (PRN) subcutaneous medication written up according to agreed guidelines.

Goal 3: discontinue inappropriate interventions.

**Psychological insight**

Goal 4: ability to communicate in English assessed as adequate.

Goal 5: insight into condition assessed.

**Religious/spiritual support**

Goal 6: religious/spiritual needs assessed with patient/carer.

**Communication**

Goal 7: identify how family/other are to be informed of patient's impending death.

Goal 8: family/other given hospital/hospice facilities leaflet.

Goal 9: GP practice is aware of patient's condition.

**Summary**

Goal 10: plan of care explained and discussed with patient/family/other.

Goal 11: family/other express understanding of care plan.

---

*Source*: Kinder and Ellershaw,[28] p. 13.

## The Gold Standards Framework for Palliative Care (GSF)

Attempts to enable primary healthcare teams (PHCT) to provide high standards of well-coordinated palliative care have been developing over the last 15 years, most notably through the work of Macmillan Cancer Relief. The Macmillan Facilitator Programme was established in 1992 in partnership with the RCGP, employing mainly practising GPs with an interest and experience in palliative care to work with their local medical colleagues in general practice to promote high standards of palliative care.[30] An evaluation of the programme found that such facilitators, who acted as a bridge between specialist and primary care in order to improve the collaboration and coordination of services, were valued by fellow GPs.[31]

The most prominent development arising from the GP facilitator programme is the GSF. The aim of the GSF is 'to develop a practice/ locally based system to improve and optimise the organisation and quality of care for patients and their carers in the last year of life'.[32] Its five objectives are to ensure:

1.  patients' symptoms are as well controlled as possible

2.  patients live and die where they choose

3.  better advanced care planning and information leads to less fear and fewer crises/admissions.

4.  carers are well supported, enabled, empowered and satisfied.

5.  staff confidence, teamworking, satisfaction and communication are improved.[32]

The GSF was developed 'from within primary care for primary care'[32] largely by Dr Keri Thomas, Macmillan GP Adviser, in 2001 following visits to over 70 practice teams and several workshops that she organised in her role as a Macmillan GP Facilitator in Palliative Care in Huddersfield, West Yorkshire. Support in the initial development was provided by a multidisciplinary reference group of specialists and generalist doctors and nurses with the aim of 'improving palliative care provided in the community by the patient's usual health care team'.[33] Phase 1 of the new framework was piloted over a period of one year in West Yorkshire with 12 practices. Each practice had a coordinator, usually a DN or alternatively the practice manager and a lead GP. Phase 1 was evaluated using a series of questionnaires, focus groups and semi-structured interviews with GPs a year after completion of the pilot.[33]

Following the success of phase 1, the GSF was expanded with the support of Macmillan Cancer Relief and the Cancer Services Collaborative of the NHS Modernisation Agency. Phase 2 was conducted with a central team to oversee the project and involved 76 practices in 18 areas. In addition to the coordinator and lead GP in every participating practice, each project area had a facilitator, most of whom were Macmillan GP facilitators or PCT cancer lead clinicians. Evaluation was by means of questionnaires at baseline and after one year. In addition a qualitative study was undertaken by the University of Huddersfield (see below).[34]

Macmillan Cancer Relief supported four more phases (phase 3–6) in 2003–5 during which a further 1350 practices in England and Northern Ireland took part and since 2005 GSF has been fully integrated with the EoLCP with increasing numbers of practices enrolling. In Scotland there is a programme that aims to offer GSF to all practices over a three-year period, with funding provided by Macmillan and the National Lottery. The GSF structure is based on a facilitator covering a single or small collection of PCTs responsible for the recruitment of practices and providing support through the set-up period. Facilitators come from a variety of backgrounds, some being GPs and others senior nurses in management roles. Participating coordinators are invited to attend three workshops during the first year of the programme and receive resource packs to offer guidance to those participating in the GSF. Practices complete questionnaires to enable feedback on their performance and monitoring of the programme centrally.

### GSF and continuity of care

Activity within the GSF focuses on seven key areas (see Box 11.3), all of which are important to aid the delivery of effective palliative care. Continuity is specifically identified as a key area (C4). For each patient the lead GP and DN is identified (*relational continuity*), plus a deputy to cover during absences. There is evidence that palliative care patients value personal continuity[35] (see Chapter 5). Maintenance of such personal relationships between patient and health professional should facilitate discussion regarding sensitive issues[35] such as preferred place of death.

All palliative care patients estimated to be in the last six to 12 months of life are identified and placed on a supportive care register that is designed to contain important, regularly updated information about the patient and to be used in care planning, thus enabling *continuity of management*. This register forms the basis of all

---

Box 11.3 **Seven key areas in primary palliative care**

---

**C1: communication**

Practices maintain a register of palliative care patients to aid in communication within the primary health care team (PHCT), especially with advanced care planning.

**C2: coordination**

A coordinator is appointed to maintain the register, arrange meetings and generally oversee the GSF process.

**C3: control of symptoms**

Holistic symptom control for each patient forms an essential part of care planning and provision.

**C4: continuity**

A key DN and GP are appointed for each patient. Communications occur with other teams involved in patient care, such as out-of-hours providers and specialist teams, by the use of faxes.

**C5: continued learning**

Practices use experiences of care for learning through, for example, Significant Event Analysis. In-house educational sessions and audits of care are used to continuously improve service delivery.

**C6: carer support**

Support for informal carers may be emotional or practical; for example, it may involve arranging night sitters or providing bereavement care.

**C7: care of the dying**

Appropriate care for the last days of life given by using, for example, the LCP.

---

*Source*: adapted from Thomas,[32] p. 6.

activity for the GSF, including being a prompt for discussion with the PHCTs. Identifying patients in this way is intended to enable a proactive approach to their care. Registers may be kept in paper form or computerised. A computer module compliant with most GP clinical systems is available to practices. GP practices may also develop their own systems, for instance listing palliative care patients on a whiteboard for all staff to view, including DNs and locum doctors.

Communicating with out-of-hours providers, for example by fax, to promote *continuity of information* is considered best practice for palliative care patients.[36] Out-of-hours practitioners delivering care will thus be provided with basic information concerning the patient to facilitate appropriate management and possibly prevent crisis admissions. Effective communication should also be maintained with secondary care services (*continuity across teams*), for example with oncology or specialist palliative care. This may involve working with these services to develop effective modes of communication regarding patients, for example on the use of patient-held records or email via the secure NHS Net to enable rapid information flow. Regular PHCT meetings aim to encourage the sharing of information regarding patients between team members (*continuity within teams*) so as to allow a proactive approach to planning and delivering care with the aim of reducing crises and potentially avoiding admissions to hospital.

### Evaluation of the GSF

The primary evaluation tool for phases 2–6 is a standard questionnaire covering all aspects of the framework (see Box 11.3). Practices complete questionnaires at baseline, at 6 months and 12 months. Questionnaires are collated and analysed for each phase of the GSF and the results reported to participating practices. Responses to the questionnaires indicate that the majority of practices establish a supportive care register early in their involvement with the GSF. Practices also report that they are becoming more proactive in areas such as team communication and care planning, for example in establishing a coordinator for palliative care and using team meetings for advanced planning for palliative care patients.

Activity in all areas (C1–7) of the GSF is reported to increase according to questionnaire results. These also indicate that the framework is effective in increasing the confidence of PHCT members in caring for terminally ill patients.[37]

In order to specifically examine the depth and variation of practice adoption of GSF, qualitative studies designed to explore these factors have formed part of the evaluation. King *et al.*[34] documented empirical findings based on interviews with doctors and nurses held in four geographical areas during phase 2 of the GSF programme. Two GSF practices were recruited from each area, thus totalling eight. These were matched with eight non-GSF practices in terms of list size, type of population served and make-up of the PHCT. Five members were interviewed from each practice including GPs (two), DNs (two) and the GSF coordinator (one). The perceived impact of GSF on palliative care services in the community was evaluated from the point of view of practitioners. Implementing GSF was found to make practices more aware of the standard of service delivery, for example with regard to the organisation of out-of-hours services. Forward planning inspired practices to take a more anticipatory approach to care, with the result that crises including admission to hospital could be avoided, for example by addressing medication needs *before* nausea and constipation reached a critical stage.

One of the key benefits of GSF cited was improved communication within the PHCT. This tended to be especially valued by DNs, who commonly report difficulties experienced in establishing good communication with GPs. District nurses tended to be more positive about the scheme than GPs because of the potential to improve communication and coordination. More GPs than DNs, however, queried whether the benefits of GSF were sufficient to warrant continued participation, given the costs in time and effort. Such attitudes were deemed to partly stem from GPs' exposure to competing demands from other primary care initiatives as practices are made subject to numerous local and national targets and priorities.

An emerging issue for some practices was not whether GSF had delivered improvements but the extent to which the merits of the programme warranted its continuation in view of the cost of time and resources, and an excessive amount of paperwork associated with the scheme. Whilst all the practices in the case studies implemented the scheme at more than a purely symbolic level, they were regarded as varying considerably in the depth of adoption and the extent to which GSF permeated the working lives of primary care staff. The study provides insight into the multiple and conflicting perspectives of GPs and DNs towards implementing GSF, and the differing levels of commitment displayed even among partners for introducing it within practices.

For phases 3–6 a case study evaluation is being undertaken that will examine the extent to which GSF has been implemented by a selection of practices, the role of the facilitator in recruiting and assisting practices in establishing GSF, and the part played by local factors such as the PCT or Cancer Network strategy, in influencing the operation of this programme. It will examine the levers and barriers to GSF implementation and provide insights for further development of the framework and community palliative care.

## Discussion

Patients with end-stage disease of any diagnosis, particularly those with complex needs and a definable terminal phase, present a challenge to all healthcare professionals. Primary care teams, especially the GP and DN, have traditionally been at the forefront of caring for these patients in the community. However, as management strategies in advanced cancer evolve, with increasing disease-modifying treatments nearer to the end of life and the widening of the multidisciplinary team,[38] primary palliative care has become more complex and challenging. Changes to primary care practice including the new GMS contract may further threaten personal continuity of care traditionally offered by many GPs.

Frameworks such as the GSF aspire to achieve continuity of care by identifying key professionals, encouraging regular meetings for patient review and advanced care planning, and ensuring the efficient flow of information to out-of-hours providers and specialist teams. It has been suggested that the GSF provides a means of enabling PHCTs to maintain one of their core values – the provision of person-centred care.[11] The spread of GSF in spite of the fact that it does not attract enhanced payments for practices may reveal the value and importance attached to the provision of patient-centred palliative care by health professionals who have persevered without much financial incentive. There is also evidence that DNs perceive the GSF as a means to ensure that GPs engage with them in a multidisciplinary approach to palliative care.[34] The PPOC tool may also provide a framework for DNs to increase their influence in caring for those with palliative needs using a patient-centred approach.

At the time of writing, the EoLCP is still within its first year of operation. The funding of this programme (approximately £100,000 per million population) is limited considering its far-reaching aims of providing 'greater choice for patients in where they want to live and die irrespective of their diagnosis'. Whether frameworks such as the GSF and PPOC tool can produce a major and sustainable improvement in palliative services in the context of a radically changing primary care landscape and limited levels of funding is unclear (see Chapter 15). It is possible, however, that such initiatives will have an indirect but positive effect on practices that are not taking a formal part, but which are influenced by publicity, the activity of neighbouring practices and the rising profile of palliative care within governmental, professional and public consciousness. Whilst many of these questions may remain unanswered in the short term, it can be asserted with confidence that the key champions who have developed these frameworks and many who are implementing them do not lack the determination, vision and passion to enhance the quality of palliative services for those approaching the closure of life.

### Acknowledgements

Prof. Scott Murray provided helpful comments on an earlier draft. Many of the issues discussed in this chapter have developed through our involvement with the Macmillan GSF Evaluation and Research Group chaired by Professor Jane Maher and Dr Keri Thomas. Many thanks to all of those involved.

---

### Summary

- The primary care team remains central to delivery of palliative care in the community.

- Increasing specialisation may lead to loss of skills for generalists.

- Patient choice over where to be cared for and die is central to good palliative care.

- The NHS End-of-Life Care Programme (EoLCP) aims to increase and empower patient choice and improve care of the dying.

- The Gold Standards Framework (GSF), Preferred Place of Care Tool (PPOC) and Liverpool Care of the Dying Pathway (LCP) are designed to ensure good practice and continuity of care.

- Reorganisation of the NHS and changes within professional and public consciousness regarding end-of-life care are likely to influence primary palliative care developments.

### REFERENCES

1. Seale C and Cartwight A. *The Year before Death.* Aldershot, Hants: Avebury, 1994.

2. Field D. Special not different: General practitioners' accounts of their care of dying people. *Social Science and Medicine* 1998; **46 (9)**: 1111–20.

3. Charlton R. Palliative care is integral to practice. *British Medical Journal* 1995; **311 (7018)**: 1503.

4. Luker K, Austin L, Caress A and Hallet C. The importance of 'knowing the patient': Community nurses' constructions of quality in providing palliative care. *Journal of Advanced Nursing* 2000; **31**: 775–82.

5. Goodman C, Knight D, Machen I and Hunt B. Emphasizing terminal care as district nurse work: A helpful strategy in a purchasing environment. *Journal of Advanced Nursing* 1998; **28**: 491–8.

6. Griffiths J. Holistic district nursing: Care for the terminally ill. *British Journal of Community Nursing* 1997; **2**: 440–4

7. McWhinney I. Primary care: Core values. Core values in a changing world. *British Medical Journal* 1998; **316**: 1807–9.

8. Heath I. The cawing of the crow … Cassandra like, prognosticating woe. *British Journal of General Practice* 2004; 54: 320–1.

9. Murray SA, Boyd K, Sheikh A, Thomas K and Higginson IJ. Developing primary palliative care. *British Medical Journal* 2004; **329 (7474)**: 1056–7.

10. Marshall M and Roland M. The new contract: Renaissance or requiem for general practice? *British Journal of General Practice* 2002; **52**: 531–2.

11. Walton W-J. The wisdom lost in knowledge: Changes in the face of general practice. *Journal of the Royal Society of Medicine* 2005; **98**: 37–8.

12. National Service Frameworks [web page]. Available at: www.dh.gov.uk/ PolicyAndGuidance/HealthAndSocialCareTopics/HealthAndSocialCareArt icle/fs/en?CONTENT_ID=4070951&chk=W3ar/W [accessed March 2007].

13. *Guidance on Cancer Services: Improving supportive and palliative care for adults.* London: National Institute for Clinical Excellence, 2004.

14. Addington-Hall J and McCarthy M. Dying from cancer: Results of a national population-based investigation. *Palliative Medicine* 1995; **9**: 295–305.

15. Townsend J, Frank A, Fermont D, *et al.* Terminal cancer care and patients' preference for place of death: A prospective study. *British Medical Journal* 1990; **301**: 415–17.

16. Higginson I, Jarman B, Astin P and Dolan S. Do social factors affect where patients die: An analysis of 10 years of cancer deaths in England. *Journal of Public Health Medicine* 1999; **21**: 22–8.

17. Grande G, Addington-Hall J and Todd C J. Place of death and access to home care services: Are certain patient groups at a disadvantage. *Social Science and Medicine* 1998; **47 (5)**: 565–79.

18. Karlsen S and Addington-Hall J. How do cancer patients who die at home differ from those who die elsewhere? *Palliative Medicine* 1998; **12**: 279–86.

19. Higginson I and Sen-Gupta GJ. Place of care in advanced cancer: A qualitative systematic literature review of patient preferences. *Journal of Palliative Medicine* 2000; **3**: 287–300.

20. Hinton J. Can home care maintain an acceptable quality of life for patients with terminal cancer and their relatives? *Palliative Medicine* 1994; **8**: 183–96.

21. Grinyer A and Thomas C. The importance of place of death in young adults with terminal cancer. *Mortality* 2004; **9**: 114–31.

22. Thomas C, Morris S and Clark D. Place of death: Preferences among cancer patients and their carers. *Social Science and Medicine* 2004; **58**: 2431–44.

23. Thomas C. The place of death of cancer patients: Can qualitative data add to known factors? *Social Science and Medicine* 2005; **60**: 2597–607.

24. Bliss J and While A. Decision-making in palliative and continuing care in the community: An analysis of the published literature with reference to the context of UK care provision. *International Journal of Nursing Studies* 2003; **40**: 881–8.

25. *Building on the Best: Choice, responsiveness and equity in the NHS.* London: Department of Health, 2003.

26. Storey L, Pemberton C, Howard A and O'Donnell L. Place of death: Hobson's choice or patient choice? *Cancer Nursing Practice* 2003; **2**: 33–8.

27. The Preferred Place of Care Plan and why it was developed [web page]. Available at: www.cancerlancashire.org.uk/ppc.html [accessed March 2007].

28. Kinder C and Ellershaw J. How to use the Liverpool Care of the Dying Pathway for the Dying Patient. In: Ellershaw J and Wilkinson S, eds. *Care of the Dying: A pathway to excellence.* Oxford: Oxford University Press, 2003, pp. 11–41.

29. Foster A, Rosser E, Kendall M and Barrow K. Implementing the Liverpool Care Pathway for the Dying Patient (LCP) in hospital, hospice, community and nursing home. In: Ellershaw J and Wilkinson S, eds. *Care of the Dying: A pathway to excellence.* Oxford: Oxford University Press, 2003. pp. 121–40.

30. How to become a Macmillan GP in England [web page]. Available at: www. macmillan.org.uk/About_Us/Source_of_support/Specialist_healthcare/ How_to_become_a_Macmillan_Health_Professional/How_to_become_a_ Macmillan_GP_in_England.aspx [accessed March 2007].

31. Shipman C, Addington-Hall J, Thompson M, *et al.* Building bridges in palliative care: Evaluating a GP facilitator programme. *Palliative Medicine* 2003; **17 (7)**: 621–7.

32. Thomas K. GSF Welcome Pack for Practice Co-ordinators and PCT Facilitators [web page]. 2005; available at: www.goldstandardsframework.nhs.uk/content/ facilitator_starter_pack/Combined_Welcom5_version_7.pdf [accessed March 2007].

33 Thomas K. *Caring for the Dying at Home: Companions on the journey.* Oxford: Radcliffe, 2003.

34. King N, Thomas K, Martin N, Bell D and Farrell S. 'Now nobody falls through the net': Practitioners' perspectives on the Gold Standards Framework for community palliative care. *Palliative Medicine* 2005; **19**: 619–27.

35. Schers H, Webster S, van den Hoogen H, Avery A, Grohl R and van den Bosch W. Continuity of care in general practice: A survey of patients' views. *British Journal of General Practice* 2002; **52**: 459–62.

36. *Raising Standards for Patients: New partnerships in out of hours care.* London: Department of Health, 2000.

37. Summary of GSF evaluation [web page]. 2005; available at: www. goldstandardsframework.nhs.uk/content/evaluation_and_research/ Macmillan_UK_Conference_19-01-05.pdf [accessed March 2007].

38. Murphy E. Case management and community matrons for long term conditions. *British Medical Journal* 2004; **329**: 1251–2.

CHAPTER | 12

# Communication in palliative care
## Patient-held records
*Michael A. Cornbleet*

---

## Introduction

'Communication, communication, communication' is an oft-repeated chant when failings of medical care are being discussed. Whether between carer and patient, patient and doctor, doctor and nurse, hospital and general practice, secondary and tertiary care, the vast number of interfaces that a patient has to negotiate in the course of any chronic condition makes communication a vital component of effective care. This is particularly exemplified by an illness such as cancer, where the 'patient journey' is complex, involves many disciplines often in several hospitals and may span a considerable length of time. It is therefore no surprise that a recent study demonstrated the problems for only one discipline when it revealed the median number of doctors encountered by patients by the time they were in a specialist palliative care setting to be 32.[1] That differing messages and interpretations confuse some patients is less of a surprise than that some patients are not confused. Failures of communication underlie much of the dissatisfaction that leads to formal complaints about health care, which might be seen as an inevitable consequence (see Chapter 5).

One of the possible means of mitigating the difficulties created by this was suggested in the study cited above and others.[2,3] The Calman–Hine report[2] saw patient-held records (PHR) as a potential answer to some of these concerns: 'Further development of PHRs, which could contain important details of the patient's management by all those involved in their care should be encouraged.' In other contexts, PHRs are well established. Examples include obstetrics,[4] child health[5] and chronic illness,[6] where moves towards greater patient involvement in their own care and decision making about that care have been demonstrated to be effective and popular. In cancer care, a number of small studies have also suggested that the development of an acceptable PHR is welcomed by patients but is not without difficulty.[7,8,9] The advantages of ready access to current information by, for example, out-of-hours medical cover and improved continuity of care might be offset by the imposition of more information than some patients might want, or health professionals be willing to provide. The other major obstacle to widespread enthusiasm amongst healthcare professionals has been the recognition of an inevitable increase in workload. No currently available format of PHR could replace the clinical records of GP, district nurse, hospital specialist(s), hospice in-patient or home-care team and so maintaining a PHR, handwritten because it needs to be current, will represent additional work and, more significantly, time. When this reservation is compounded by the discomfort some (particularly doctors) will feel about the degree of openness, patient participation and honest discussion of prognosis that would be necessary, the idea begins to look much less attractive. The GP may need to know as soon as possible that the liver function tests or ultrasound appearances are worsening. However, that information can't be handwritten in a PHR by a specialist nurse or consultant unless they have (and are willing to make available there and then) the time to explain what the implications of those findings are. If not, the patient or carer will read them at home without immediate recourse to explanation or support. A further belief is that by no means every patient will welcome the greater degree of involvement, and that having such a record at home might have the effect of the illness/hospital intruding into the 'sanctuary' of home. The two roles proposed for PHRs, as a tool for patients' empowerment and information or as a means of interprofessional communication, are not difficult to see coming into conflict if the solution is a single document.

### The Scottish trial

The traditional means of approaching a problem such as this is the randomised controlled trial, and such a trial has been conducted for the use of a PHR in cancer/palliative care.[10] This study was commissioned by the Joint Working Party on Patient-Held Records of the Scottish Partnership for Palliative Care and the National Council for Hospice and Specialist Palliative Care Services. Evidence considered by the working party showed that PHRs that had been developed in a variety of clinical settings shared many common features, but that their development had been time consuming. The duplication of effort led this study, as a deliberate policy, to utilise a model of patient-held record developed after exhaustive consultation and discussion over a two-year period, but in a different area of the country and with a slightly different patient population.[11] Patients were recruited into a prospective, parallel group, randomised controlled trial from oncology out-patient clinics or hospice home-care or day-care settings in the central belt in Scotland. Two hundred and forty-four patients were randomised and 231 completed the baseline interview. One hundred and seventeen were randomised to have the PHR and 114 to the control group receiving standard care. At the follow-up interview six months later, 80 patients in the PHR group and 97 in the control group were available for interview. The main outcome measures were the subjective views of patient satisfaction with communication and perception of communication between patient and healthcare professionals, as determined by structured interview conducted by an independent observer. A postal opinion survey of 83 health professionals known to have received the PHR was conducted 14 months into the study and received 63 replies.

The groups were similar in all significant demographic characteristics at the outset of the study and in their levels of information and satisfaction with communication. Two-thirds of patients in both groups described themselves as satisfied or very satisfied with information provided by hospital staff. At follow-up, no improvement in the provision of information or patient satisfaction with information provided by out-patient doctors, primary care teams or hospice staff could be identified. Overall, patients' perceptions of communication between all staff involved in their care either with or without a PHR was excellent in 24 per cent and 21 per cent respectively, or very good in 56 per cent and 58 per cent ($p = 0.89$). The PHR made no difference to information passing between health professional or to the degree of family involvement. However, while those who had and used a PHR spoke highly of it (indeed, sometimes in almost euphoric terms), a significant minority (14 per cent) did not use it and 20 per cent identified features they disliked, such as the additional perceived responsibility and having to ask health professionals to complete it. Of the health professionals responding to the postal survey, 73 per cent said they were aware that their patient had a PHR, but only a third of respondents felt that all of their patients with a PHR offered it to them, while 16 per cent never did so. Only 35 per cent of hospital staff said that they had asked for the record, whereas 68 per cent of staff in the community had done so, clearly contributing to the impression that the onus was on the patient to produce and ensure completion of the record. Although undoubtedly a reassuring finding, the high initial level of satisfaction at the outset limited the scope for improvement that could be achieved by the PHR and reduced the statistical power of the study.

**The problems**

Problems identified by the authors included the anticipated lack of local ownership. It is difficult to know the extent to which this coloured the attitudes of health professionals, but the very extensive consultation that preceded its development in Newcastle over a two-year period must have developed a strong local commitment to using the final product.[11] Although considerable effort was made to explain and introduce the study to all who were to participate, this did not establish a sufficient sense of ownership when compared with the additional work that was anticipated. And this was an obstacle that could not be overcome. All the professionals in the study had to maintain their own records and none felt able to diminish either the quality or quantity of those records in favour of entries in the PHR. They were therefore not consistently used except by patients who used them essentially as diaries that, while of considerable value, did not provide the professional carers with the information they thought they could expect. As soon as the record could not be relied on to be accurate and current, it lost most of its utility for the health professionals, and once they ceased asking for it patients became reluctant to ask them to write in it.

It is also of interest to note that, when asked whether they would be willing to implement a PHR for routine use, only slightly more than half answered in the affirmative, but half the doctors did not respond regarding those with advanced cancer. A substantial minority of nurses responded negatively or did not respond.

The practice of modern medicine, perhaps in particular oncology and palliative care, involves the acquisition and interpretation of enormous volumes of data. Appropriate decision making about treatment options available at different points in the journey depend on this information being available in the right place and at the right time. Further, it needs to be made understandable to the patient and carers if they are to be meaningfully enabled to participate in decisions about their treatment and care. In this context, the appeal of a patient-held record is obvious, but the many pitfalls identified in the Scottish study and others[11,12] suggest that further questions need to be asked before assuming that the widespread adoption of a PHR will solve these problems. First, if it is indeed the case that local ownership is central to the general and consistent utilisation of a PHR, there will inevitably be much duplication of effort. There is good evidence that local enthusiasm is perhaps the single most important determination of success, but the expense of time and effort if replicated in every cancer and palliative care team would be prohibitive. The final product in each area will inevitably look similar, but, crucially, not identical. The PHR used in Scotland was modified with local information wherever appropriate, but was still perceived as derived from elsewhere. Second, and more fundamentally, the divergence of functionality between what a patient wants and what a health professional needs may be impossible to resolve in a single document. The details of the latest blood count of a patient undergoing chemotherapy may be essential to the proper assessment of a febrile patient by an out-of-hours doctor called at 3 a.m., but requires a different functionality from the recording by the patient of pain or nausea if it is be useful.

**The future?**

It is possible that the long-awaited improvements in information management technology within the NHS will take the debate into new areas. In areas where technology is already routinely making current patient information available simultaneously to primary and secondary care, pilot studies are underway to assess the value of a printout formatted to the patient's needs to be provided to them as a PHR. Such work is underway in diabetes care, where parameters of glycaemia control such as HbAIc and cholesterol can be printed out and maintained in a ring binder or other appropriate form. However, in such a system, the information printed out is already directly accessible in a GP surgery, as they can access the same laboratory system, so the 'added value' needs to be assessed. In addition, the ways that patients will use such information need to be determined. If they choose to use the 'patient diary' element of such a record, do health professionals read it and act on the content? If not, will it cause anger and frustration? It may, however, turn out that the main benefit of such systems is that time no longer needed to transmit routine information between health professionals is made available for real and meaningful discussion with a patient or carer, and that would probably impact more on patient (and professional) satisfaction and effectiveness of care than any format of PHR could reasonably expect to.

---

## Summary

- Patient-held records need to fill a clearly specified role.

- Local ownership and enthusiasm are critical to utilisation.

- Patients and clinicians need to understand the distinction between clinical record and patient diary functions.

- Not every patient will want, or benefit, from a patient-held record.

---

REFERENCES

1. Smith SDM, Nicol KM, Devereux J and Cornbleet MA. Encounters with doctors: Quantity and quality? *Palliative Medicine* 1999; **13**: 217–23.

2. Expert Advisory Group on Cancer to the Chief Medical Officers of England and Wales. *A Policy Framework for Commissioning Cancer Services* [the 'Calman/Hine Report']. London: Department of Health, 1995.

3. Scottish Cancer Co-ordinating Committee. *Commissioning Cancer Services in Scotland: Primary and palliative care services. Report to the Chief Medical Officer.* Edinburgh: SODoH, 1997.

4. Lovell A, Zander L, James C, *et al.* The St Thomas's Hospital maternity case notes study: A randomised controlled trial to assess the effects of giving expectant mothers their own maternity case notes. *Paediatric and Perinatal Epidemiology* 1987; **1**: 57–66.

5. Macfarlane A. Personal child health records held by parents. *Archives of Disease in Childhood* 1992; **67(5)**: 571–2.

6. Essex B, Doig R and Renshaw J. Pilot study of records of shared care for people with mental illness. *British Medical Journal* 1990; **300**: 1442–6.

7. Dougherty L and Stuttaford J. Turning over a new leaflet. *Nursing Times* 1996; **89**: 46–8.

8. Hayward K. Patient-held oncology records. *Nursing Standard* 1998; **12**: 44–6.

9. Drury M, Harcourt J and Minton M. The acceptability of patients with cancer holding their own shared-care record. *Psycho-Oncology* 1996; **5**: 119–25.

10. Cornbleet MA, Campbell P, Murray S, Stevenson M and Bond S. Patient-held records in cancer and palliative care: A prospective, randomised trial. *Palliative Medicine* 2002; **16**: 205–12.

11. Lecouturier J, Crack L, Mannix K, Hall R and Bond S. *Care to Communicate? Evaluating a patient-held record for patients with cancer.* Report No 102. Newcastle: Centre for Health Services Research, University of Newcastle, 1999.

12. Finlay IG and Wyatt P. Randomised cross-over study of patient-held records in oncology and palliative care. *Lancet* 1999; **353**: 558–9.

CHAPTER | 13

# Communication in palliative care

## IT systems

*Max Watson*

---

## Introduction

The world of palliative care, in common with most other clinical areas, seems to be divided between those who have tremendous enthusiasm for computers and the benefits of information technology (IT) – *technophiles* – and those who are not and see computerisation as yet another barrier between healthcare professionals and patients in need of quality holistic care – *technophobes* (see Box 13.1). Both mindsets can affect the quality, of care that a palliative team can provide for their patients.

---

### Box 13.1 **The technophile and the technophobe**

The *technophile* can become so engrossed in developing the ultimate software package that will monitor every bowel motion and DS1500 application that he or she ends up skimping on his or her clinical workload. He or she prefers to spend time with 'virtual' patients rather than with real ones, who seldom fit into the computerised boxes that they should.

Such an approach is quickly noticed by the rest of the team, who not only have difficulty understanding some of his or her IT enthusiasm but are aware that their clinical workload is increased by a team member spending hours before his or her computer.

The *technophobe* has frequently been inoculated by the 'virus' of computer incompetence. This virus conveys a deep-seated distrust of the electronic, a distrust that may mask a genuine fear of being trapped in a job where he or she has to face up to learning how to use a computer.

Stories about long-dead patients being sent invitations for dental appointments and gas bills for millions of pounds are an ongoing defence against the day when he or she may have to face his or her antipathy to electronic technology and learn.

---

Both technophobe and technophile share an approach to IT that elevates it from its true role as a tool for dealing with information efficiently and quickly to a quasi-mystical force worthy of veneration or hatred.

In devising appropriate strategies for using information technology in palliative care it is important not to begin with leaflets about the latest computer or dedicated software package. Installing a computer system is expensive and the system is likely to be worthless unless it is accompanied by:

- a clear understanding of what the team hopes to gain from computerisation
- whether such aspirations are feasible with available and affordable systems
- which system is the best option
- a clear programme for training of staff
- and clearly set targets for the gradual introduction of a system.

It is also important to review, perhaps by way of a formal audit, how well the existing *system* is functioning and how that system is meeting the needs of patients and team members. If your team has an existing inefficient information system, it is unlikely that computerising that system will do anything other than highlight the deficiencies and confirm the technophobe's deepest held suspicions about computers

## IT systems for palliative care

Information technology in palliative care can be extremely valuable in a number of ways. It can:

- help deliver quality care to patients and families in an auditable fashion
- allow patient care to be monitored efficiently
- share information effectively among healthcare professionals, the patient and the family
- be sensitive to the requirements of patient confidentiality and the Data Protection Act
- encourage the team to review and assess changes in its performance

- promote good working relationships
- encourage appropriate team support
- provide the information needed for meeting administrative, financial and organisational planning.

The goal is an efficient information system that serves your teams' needs, not an information system that your team must serve. Personal and repeated experience in many healthcare settings enforces the belief that computerisation is likely to be a much more rewarding process if it involves a system that is already working well. Computers will not sort out your information system problems, but they can facilitate and maximise the benefits of efficient systems.

A useful first step involves analysing the existing team information system to work out the issues. This provides a framework within which both the technophobe and technophile can look at how their team is working and face up to difficulties within the existing delivery of service and management of information. This approach earths issues in the practical realities of daily working life and can highlight practical solutions to information problems. Communication can be improved without recourse to IT and it is important that these issues are resolved in addition to commissioning computer systems (Box 13.2).

---

Box 13.2 **Non-IT solutions to communication problems**

Working as a specialist community palliative care nurse, Paula was shocked to find, when she analysed her week, that nearly 55 per cent of her time was spent answering 'phone calls or trying to contact other healthcare professionals'. In particular this was causing constant interruption to her work with patients when on home visits.

By using the palliative care secretary to handle the calls and by arranging to contact the secretary at set times during each day, Paula was able to improve her working efficiency, reduce interruptions and decrease wasted phone time.

---

## Clinical IT systems, community palliative care teams and continuity of care

Sharing information for those providing 'on call' cover can be particularly problematic. Lack of up-to-date information can make it difficult for health professionals working out of hours to make effective and safe management decisions. Computerised records enable patient details to be rapidly accessed. Records of all 'active' patients can be downloaded onto a laptop computer or handheld device – known as a personal digital assistant (PDA). The whole active patient database can then be taken home and is available if a call is received at night or when out of the office on a visit.

Alternatively the team can carry a handheld device such as a 'Blackberry', which would allow them to access the central database directly through the internet-surfing capacity of the device. With appropriate security controls and firewalls in effect this would provide every team member with the capacity to view the details of any patient on the central database, and to update that database remotely with details of patient visits. Such systems can help to ensure that patients who have particular palliative care needs and who contact the service for advice out of hours are treated appropriately.

By being thus able to update the patient electronic record remotely, even if a call occurs out of hours, important and current information is captured and made available to the rest of the team. Paper records can be unavailable through being on a desk waiting to be updated, locked in the boot of a car, misfiled in the team's storage system or lost in transit between the hospital and community palliative care team. IT records can be accessed from anywhere where the IT system is available by any team member with access rights, normally through a user code and password. Furthermore, IT records are less likely to be lost in filing.

Databases are easy to search and interrogate. Audits that would take weeks to perform by 'pulling' paper records can be completed in a matter of minutes with a computerised system. The activity profile of the palliative care team both for the healthcare professional individually, and also for the team as a whole is automatically updated and becomes almost a by-product of a properly kept clinical IT system. Being able to audit such activity is extremely valuable since increasingly this information is necessary for evaluation purposes and also to justify programmes that are under threat because of budgetary restraints and competing services.

Common problems arise with IT systems. Team members need to type their notes and this can be time consuming. If paper records are also kept 'double data entry' is a particularly lengthy and frustrating process. An alternative to healthcare professionals entering data is dictation, which a secretary can enter onto the system. This is often not feasible through lack of secretarial resources.

Patient confidentiality is a concern with any clinical IT system. By making such databases easily available to healthcare professionals who have legitimate access, there is a potential risk of inappropriate access unless secure safeguards are in place. Confidentiality can be maintained through appropriate systems of user name and password protection, and through using secure networks such as the NHS Net. With the new national IT programme for the NHS, staff will be issued with 'smart cards' that will be necessary to access the NHS Net, further increasing security. It is the responsibility of system developers to ensure that systems cannot easily be 'hacked' into and professionals need to adhere closely to policies of keeping passwords private and not leaving machines unattended if breeches of confidentiality are to be avoided. In addition, any users of computer systems to store information about individuals need to be aware of and comply with the Data Protection and Freedom of Information Acts (see Box 13.3).

---

Box 13.3 **Maintenance of privacy using biometric verification**

Recognised 'thumbprints' will allow the user to open up the computer to gain access to patient records. If the device is tampered with, or if someone with an unrecognised thumbprint tries to gain access more than three times, the data will automatically be cleared from the storage disc.

---

## Practical arrangements for using a clinical IT system in palliative care

A clinical database that contains the details of all the patients who are currently cared for by the palliative care team may be stored on a computer in the main team office, and an updated back-up copy saved to a central computer within the PCT where a regulated back-up procedure takes place.

Each night the specialist palliative care nurses update their personal PDA from the main database. Thus each nurse responsible for providing on-call cover can access up-to-date patient information quickly during the night if he or she is contacted about a patient whom he or she doesn't know.

During the night if the nurse is contacted about any patient he or she will document details of the contact in the patient's record on the PDA.

The next morning when he or she reconnects her device to the main system, it will automatically update the main database. The system could be programmed to generate a list of all the patients whom he or she has seen, or been in contact with, overnight with details of what he or she has done. This list can then be distributed to the patient's key palliative care nurse either in electronic or paper form and a copy of the same information emailed to the patient's GP.

Each of the members of the team carries their own PDA, into which they record details of all patient contacts, throughout the day. Every day they update their PDA from the central database and download to the database their own details of all patient contacts, visits and phone calls.

This system allows patient records to be:

- kept up to date
- readily accessible to team members
- auditable
- and shared with other appropriate professionals who would otherwise have to be 'phoned'.

A variation of this system would involve the nurses using remote access, e.g. with a 'Blackberry' device, to interrogate the main database and to input data directly without having to be 'in the office'. This increases flexibility but also raises issues of security. Systems managers would want to ensure that there was a high standard of data entry from the team, before opening the gates to the main database too widely.

Once a month the secretary produces the team's data sheet detailing a list of the patients who have been seen, when they have been seen, who has seen them, and what actions have been taken.

The database is very useful in producing the team's annual report for the local PCT as the secretary is able to generate the figures documenting the team's workload.

### A vision of how information handling could facilitate one patient's palliative care journey

Mr Brown, a 73-year-old married former carpenter with advanced prostate cancer, is referred to the community palliative care team by his general practitioner.

Before his first meeting the secretary initiates a new case record for Mr Brown on the palliative care database, entering all of his registration details and an electronic copy of the referral letter to the team that has been emailed over the NHS Net by the GP.

At the out-patient appointment with Mr and Mrs Brown further details are taken and entered into his electronic file.

Prior to Mr Brown leaving the clinic he is given a letter detailing the key areas covered during the consultation as well as the agreed plan and details of how to contact the palliative care team, when to contact them, and an appointment time for his next clinic.

A copy of this letter, which was generated from the information gathered at the interview, with Mr Brown's permission will also be sent to his GP, either electronically by encrypted email, or by post.

Initially nurses were very concerned that this would slow down their work. At the beginning it was very slow because the nurses didn't trust the system and as well as recording everything electronically into their PDAs they were also continuing to keep their written diaries. After a couple of months this stopped as confidence in the electronic system increased and the benefits of it were seen.

(JR, palliative care clinical nurse specialist)

Mrs Brown calls the emergency palliative care team at 2 a.m. to say that her husband is having increasing pain in his right shoulder and cannot sleep.

The on-call nurse, who does not know Mr Brown, opens his electronic record chart on her PDA and checks his details and management. She sees that he is known to have a painful metastatic bone lesion in his right shoulder. She also sees which medications he is currently taking.

As the pain is not new, but a steadily deteriorating one, the nurse advises Mrs Brown to give her husband an extra dose of his analgesic breakthrough medication, and to arrange to see his GP in the morning.

The team member records the contact in Mr Brown's electronic file.

This will generate a letter to Mr Brown's GP that will be sent electronically next morning.

### Out-patient clinic

At his palliative medicine clinic appointment 10 days later the consultant can see the interactions that have taken place and the changes to medicine made by the palliative care team. This helps her to assess his changing pain needs, which she feels could be improved by local radiotherapy to his arm. She speaks to an oncology colleague and an appointment is made for later that week.

Using the referral module, which is a standard part of the system, the consultant is able to quickly draw up a referral letter containing the key details and the reason for referral as well as current medications and give it to the patient to take. (A further copy is sent to the GP.)

### Hospice

Mr Brown's condition deteriorates and he is admitted to the hospice for symptom control. As the hospice uses the same system and database as the community palliative care team, prior to admitting Mr Brown the hospice doctor and nurse are able to access Mr Brown's full record and see exactly what has occurred with his care up until the time of admission.

When Mr Brown's pain is better controlled he is discharged home. At discharge the hospice doctor and nurse complete the electronic discharge form that includes a record of the admission, treatment changes and follow-up plans. This is emailed to his GP and hard copy printed out and sent to the oncologist for his hospital record, which is not computerised.

### Terminal phase

Mr Brown continues to weaken and in keeping with his expressed wishes he is nursed at home. He lapses into unconsciousness.

On the night before he dies, the on-call nurse is contacted by the emergency doctor on call. The doctor had had a phone call from Mr

Brown's son who was very concerned that his father seemed to be having chest problems. The son was keen that his father be admitted to the local hospital. Prior to visiting, the doctor wanted to check whether Mr Brown had recorded his wishes with regard to place of death. The nurse is able to call up the chart and find that Mr Brown had expressed the clear wish that he wanted to die at home. Accessing this information greatly helps the doctor managing the fraught situation at the Browns' home and prevents an unnecessary and potentially distressing admission through the local casualty department.

### Bereavement

Mr Brown dies the following morning and his death is recorded into the database. The database also includes details of those members of the family who will be most affected by the death.

Two months later the database generates an invitation to the bereavement evening that is held each month at the hospice.

### Audit

As part of an audit project looking at speed of communication with general practitioners, patient files, including Mr Brown's file, over a three-month period are analysed electronically, and it is found that over 95 per cent of patient contacts are reported to the GP within two working days.

### Service planning

In a bid to encourage the local PCT to employ another full-time specialist palliative care community nurse the team administrator uses the database to show how much the team's workload has increased over the previous two years, and in particular how the opening of two large residential nursing homes in the area has increased the demand for palliative care services.

While such information would have been available under the previous system, the speed of accessing the data has greatly improved. In addition, because logging contacts, visits and phone calls has become second nature to the team a far more accurate and comprehensive account of the team's workload is now being recorded and updated.

### Steps to successfully establishing a clinical IT system in community palliative care

Establishing an effective clinical IT system is complicated and potentially problematic with many foreseen and unforeseen pitfalls. It takes time, planning and patience. Personnel need to be trained and some will need more support and encouragement than others. Realistic goals within a sensible time-frame need to be set and it should be remembered that it will probably take much longer to establish than anticipated. Finally, progress needs to be regularly reviewed.

1. Review existing information system *as a team*.

2. Set out clear goals of what changes in the information system *the team* want to achieve, both in the short term but also over a five-year period.

3. Implement changes to the existing system to improve its accuracy and efficiency in line with the established goals.

4. Run the improvements for a one- to two-month period. If the changes do not meet the team's information system goals, continue to maintain the best information system possible while considering more radical alternatives.

5. Meet together as a team to decide if investing the time and resources in a more radical change in information handling is a current priority.

6. Appoint an IT lead team (ideally involving at least one technophile and one technophobe) with responsibility and dedicated time to research the various possibilities and report back to the team. Invite a member of the PCT IT department to join the group but make sure that the clinical need drives the IT development and not vice versa. Setting up systems that work requires a commitment of time and resources that need to be accounted for. Systems produced by enthusiasts in the early hours of the morning have

less chance of succeeding as they tend to have too much unbalanced investment from one enthusiast.

7. Visit other community palliative care teams and review the information systems that they are operating. There are several commercial packages on the market devised to handle the needs of community palliative care and hospices. Would such a system suit your team's needs and budget? Could an existing system be modified to suit your needs?

8. Consult with your PCT and local hospitals on their future IT strategy.

- The UK government has very ambitious IT plans regarding electronic patient-held records. However, at the same time in many health authorities even the simple transfer of information between hospitals and general practices, or clinics, has not yet been achieved.
- Such contrary views of IT reality cause confusion and disheartenment as a utopian IT ideal meets the reality of system incompatibility, bureaucracy, data protection and an NHS IT workforce who are regularly being 'headhunted' by the more lucrative private sector.
- Adopt a pragmatic approach to this tension:
  - □ the ideal system does not exist
  - □ waiting for the utopia will involve a very long wait
  - □ being aware of imminent IT changes in your PCT that help you to maximise the potential benefits of the computerisation strategy.
  - □ accept that no sooner have you established a system that inevitably another better and cheaper system, with greater features, and more compatibility will become available

9. Budget for the introduction of a new information system in terms of time, staff training, data input, implications for ongoing workload, and potential need for additional staff support during the setting up process. (As a rule of thumb if you think on initial analysis it should take X months to establish a new system, it may take up to double the time of your estimate.)

10. When drawing up the budget think also of the ongoing costs of maintaining such a system including:
    - software licence
    - maintenance contract
    - regular system updating
    - training for staff

11. Before starting staff training ensure that the central database is as accurate and as user friendly as possible, and that the secretarial staff are trained and comfortable with the new system. This will allow those being trained on the system, who may not be as used to computers, to see quickly the benefits. Alternatively, if the database is inaccurate, and not user friendly, the team could be easily frustrated.

12. Selecting a good and patient teacher of the system is crucial. Though much of the teaching will actually be carried out among the team as team members ask each other 'How did you do that?'

13. During the set-up period quick access to a source of help to answer questions is vital, and needs to be budgeted for.

14. Once training has been completed the team should set a date for going live on the new system. At the same time a review meeting should be arranged for the end of the week at which the problems of the first week will be discussed, and the team asked to keep a note of their problems.

15. Hold the review meeting with IT personnel present to help answer queries and suggestions for improvement.

16. Organise a team celebration in recognition of the birth of the new system and the increased work that the birth will have caused everyone.

17. At the end of the first month ensure that all members of the team get to see their workload figures, and the data that the system has been able to collect.

---

Box 13.4 **The Data Protection Act 1998 – a summary**

Key points to note:

- Personal data must be obtained fairly and lawfully.

- The act covers personal data in both electronic form and manual form (e.g. paper files, card indices) if the data are held in a relevant, structured filing system.

- Personal data must be kept accurate and up to date, and shall not be kept for longer than is necessary.

- Appropriate security measures must be taken against unlawful or unauthorised processing of personal data and against accidental loss of, or damage to, personal data. These include both technical measures, e.g. data encryption and the regular backing up of data files, and organisational measures, e.g. staff data protection training.

- Personal data shall not be transferred to a country outside the European Economic Area unless specific exemptions apply (e.g. if the data subject has given consent). This includes the publication of personal data on the internet.

**Data subject rights**

The act gives significant rights to individuals in respect of personal data held about them by data controllers. These include the rights:

- to make a subject access request – an individual is entitled to be supplied with a copy of all personal data held

- to prevent processing likely to cause damage or distress

- to prevent processing for the purposes of direct marketing

- to take action for compensation if they suffer damage by any contravention of the act by the data controller

- to take action to rectify, block, erase or destroy inaccurate data, and

- to request the Data Protection Commissioner to make an assessment as to whether any provision of the act has been contravened.

*Source*: www.dataprotection.gov.uk.

---

**Summary**

- Effective communication systems are more important than the latest IT software.

- IT can be an effective tool to aid communication.

- Remote access to the clinical database can aid out-of-hours continuity.

- IT provides a powerful tool for clinical and service audit.

- Effective confidentiality can be maintained using accredited clinical IT systems and by attention to detail.

- Planning for IT should be thorough, using a stepwise approach and not underestimating the time needed.

- Sequential steps to effective planning and implementation are suggested.

---

### FURTHER READING

- *ABC of Health Informatics* – a collection of 12 review articles in the *British Medical Journal*. Consecutive weeks from 10 September 2005.

### RECENT ARTICLES OF INTEREST

- Elfrink EJ, van der Rijt CC, van Boxtel RJJ, *et al.* Problem solving by telephone in palliative care: Use of a predetermined assessment tool within a program of home care technology. *Journal of Palliative Care* 2002; **18 (2)**: 105–10.

- Hughes RA. Clinical practice in a computer world: Considering the issues. *Journal of Advanced Nursing* 2003; **42 (4)**: 340–6.

- Lesage P and Portenoy RK. Ethical challenges in the care of patients with serious illness. *Pain Medicine* 2001; **2 (2)**: 121–30.

- Lind L and Karlsson D. A system for symptom assessment in advanced palliative home healthcare using digital pens. *Medical Informatics and the Internet in Medicine* 2004; **29 (3–4)**: 199–210.

- Quan KH, Vigano A and Fainsinger RL. Evaluation of a data collection tool (TELEform) for palliative care research. *Journal of Palliative Medicine* 2003; **6 (3)**: 401–8.

### WEBSITES

- National Programme for IT in the NHS □ www.connectingforhealth.nhs.uk/ □ (the website of NpFIT – all NHS developments in IT will be linked to this project).

- National Council for Palliative Care □ www.ncpc.org.uk/ □ (section on the Minimum Data Set for Palliative Care – IT systems should collect this information as a minimum).

- Palliative Care Matters □ www.pallcare.info/ □ (useful palliative care material including links to other sources on the internet).

CHAPTER | 14

# Ethical issues in providing continuity in palliative care

*Rob George*

Not so long ago in a galaxy very close by, doctors were entirely autonomous and effectively unimpeachable for they 'knew' what was 'best' for 'their' patients. GPs 'owned' their patient lists, often cared for individuals from cradle to grave and referred to consultants whom they knew personally or were at their *alma mater*. Doctor knew best, and consultants knew best of all. The certainty of that knowledge fell with status like a prophetic mantle and assumed pontifical proportions in teaching hospitals. Allied healthcare professionals were the handmaidens and footmen of these beneficent fiefdoms and social services seldom crossed the radar except to take the blame for bed-blockers. The GP was a pillar of the community, but continuity in secondary care was at best seeing the same doctor twice. As for continuity across the primary–secondary interface, admitting registrars will recall the standard GP letter 'Please see and do the necessary' and, if lucky, the GP may get a cryptic note a fortnight after discharge.

Whilst thankfully now generally dead, the attitudes of demigods still remain, as Nietzsche would have it, 'in some caves'. However, society, medical education and the NHS's modernisation agenda are actively enforcing structures and accountabilities that will make engagement with one's ethical duties inescapable. The question to consider is what these may be in relation to continuity of care (CoC). I am taking it as given, of course, that it is a good idea when caring for patients with complex or chronic problems for professionals to communicate and collaborate in case management. This for me is the purpose of continuity of care.

This chapter covers an extensive and complex area, and has two main purposes: first to lay out the ethical landscape in which CoC must operate and, second, to offer a practical means to resolve conflicts. Since each can be seen as separate, the two sections can be read alone. In the first, I frame the principles, problems and challenges of making increasingly complex care effective, efficient and economical. The second (comprising two parts) outlines the method and application of practical reasoning based around cases that show typical areas of difficulty in continuity.

## FRAMING THE PROBLEM

### The environment of care

This is a time of rapid change in health and social care with two issues running parallel: on the one hand an increasing emphasis on autonomy and on the other a recognition that the financial burdens of health care are rising with the age of the population. The challenge of fair and appropriate distribution of increasingly scarce resources is real. In other words, the battle between consumerism and utility is on.

### *The principle and scope of autonomy*

Definition
Most concisely stated, autonomy is 'the ability to choose, and the freedom to choose, between competing conceptions of how we live'[1] (*auto* – self and *nomon* – rule or custom). In the 'developed world', within the structure of *prima-facie* (literally on first blush or sight) freedoms and entitlements, it is increasingly unassailable. For example, in applying the principle of autonomy, the interests of a person are defined by them – a person's best interest is what they say it is. These interests do not have to be rational or beneficial according to another's view. They are simply what the individual considers them to be. This is perfectly reasonable as a cardinal *principle* since the individual is the basic brick of a free society and therefore respect for his or her autonomy is one cornerstone. However, things cannot stop there as it is equally clear and fundamental that limit has to be set to one's self-determination with self-government (personal restraint),

or law, in order to preserve the freedoms of others. Broadly speaking, though, autonomy framed as self-determination is the trump in matters of agreed individual freedoms (and the freedom to refuse treatments is principal amongst these)[2] but falls short of the right to demand whatever one wants.[3]

### Application

It takes little reflection to realise that the need for a concept of autonomy only comes when people are in relationship or community, i.e. when one has to take account of another when deciding what to do. In other words, the very idea of autonomy only takes seed because the individual's desires must be limited for the sake of others.

The practical, clinical applications of respect for the autonomy are:

1. the presumption that a patient is competent to make decisions about his or her care until proven otherwise

2. to ensure that information is adequate, comprehensible and accurate, and that sufficient opportunity has been given to discussion and weighing of options

3. to ensure that confidentiality is preserved, and

4. to ensure that the patient has consented to a plan of action.

This is how one ought to formulate and implement a competent patient's best interests and is of course the ethical basis for a form of teamwork that recognises not only the need for diverse professional contributions to understanding and responding to a patient's need, but also the inclusion of the patient as an integral part of that team.

In the pursuit of the principle of autonomy, this role for the patient is also being extended beyond the time of his or her capacity with new legislation. In 2007, the Mental Capacity Act 2005[4] (MCA) will come into force. First, this gives legal force to valid advance statements (living wills) made by the patient when capable. Second, the status of *designated* family or friends will change. Clinicians are of course acutely aware of the influence that family may wield in care and decision making already. Under the MCA, should a patient become incapable, in the absence of a valid advance statement, legal authority is extended to individuals granted lasting powers of attorney, or court-appointed deputies, to take decisions in health care and represent views on behalf of the incapable patient.[4,5] I will return to this matter in the cases since the MCA is fundamentally relevant to CoC.

### Choice versus utility

The bottom line on autonomy is that a patient's freedom or negative right to refuse, if valid and specific, is inviolable. What now of a patient's entitlements or positive rights? Whilst the *idea* of individuals having the final say in their destiny is laudable and proper, and rights are taken to be limitless by the *vox pop*, we live in an imperfect world of relationships where there is a need to codify areas of legitimate self-determination and entitlements, and areas of necessary self-government.

Entitlements
For the time being at least, citizens are entitled to free health care provided that it is recognised by society as a need. Since the national budget for health is finite, this list of needs must also be so. Therefore, the *reality* of choice over what, how and where care will take place – and this is the substance of continuity of care – is also limited. Nevertheless, the rhetoric of choice continues to influence government policy and finds its current form in the plans for patient-led commissioning and the developing framework of payment by results. (This is the current idea that specific packets of health benefit are matched by standardised and costed packets of health resource. Clearly this opens up a currency for any provider, public or private, to offer certain Health Resource Groups. However, this approach is this year's answer. To define or predict the gymnastics of NHS politics is a fool's errand and will continue well beyond the useful life of this publication.)

What is inescapable is that the future remains open given the change in British demographics and privatisation will become increasingly likely in coming decades. In these circumstances, patients will call the tune in the delivery of their needs and wants because they will pay the piper, whilst, no doubt, continuity will be orchestrated by us.

Until then the continuity of a person's care is determined by a complex calculus of competing obligations by service providers to tailor care to the individual within the strictures of resource, the pressures of increasingly costly and complex regimes, and the legitimate needs of others. Effective relationships and packages of care that hold to the principle of autonomy and the restraints of utility boil down to respect for the individual in an environment of reality.

### The practical elements of defining utility

Moving to the reality of care, one operates in the tension of the immediate duty to the patient and the obligation to offer the best achievable care for the greatest number in order to optimise cost (economic utility), convenience and efficiency (practical utility), and safety (governance). Whilst we aspire to fulfil every patient's wishes, this can only be an aspiration for all. For example, whilst desirable, the reality of providing care in the home for the severely disabled or demented may be impractical or unachievable in some patients without prohibitive financial, civil or personal cost.

---

**Box 14.1  The centrality of autonomy in care**

The centrality of autonomy in care is expressed in the facts that:

- Patients may say no to recommended actions, and, provided they are capable, that is it.

- We are obliged to operate within the tension of what people want and what resources dictate that they can have (defined by society increasingly through legislation and 'evidence-based guidance', and expressed as *need*).

- In terms of the counter to requests or demands by patients, professionals cannot refuse on the basis of best interest, as has been the historical view, for the patient is the custodian of his or her interests as a free citizen. However, in the context of the principle of autonomy, the autonomy of others (including professionals) does stand, and forms the brake or limit to the individual by society.

---

Hence, society must set limits to entitlements. In simple terms, these limits ensure that a society deals with its citizens justly. Hence, entitlements are allocated or available according to what is fair (what one deserves) and equitable (appropriate) based on a starting point of equality. The most obvious connection of these general points to CoC is in the cost and choice of places of care in the chronically sick, and in managing care where a patient refuses recommendations by professionals.

Community versus institution

Generally speaking, concentrating expertise and provision is the pragmatic solution to limited human and financial resources. In situations where acute or specialist care is the need, institutions are the solution, provided they are used for their purpose to justify cost. Where continuing care is the issue, in-patient care is simpler to implement and administer, and by and large is cheaper than care at home. This of course may be seen by the patient as his or her best interest if he or she recognises that independence is fading and best promoted in the safety of a care home.

For both, the potential *ethical* cost will be the full liberty of the individual for the benefit of effective resource allocation and the maintenance of continuity in care. The respect for autonomy should be consistent in its principles regardless of the setting or financial strictures. I will consider how this is expressed through professionals' respective duties of care next, but, first, mention must be made of two issues: the philosophical tension that fuels the historical antipathy between health and social services to form the conflicting views of the purpose of care. Second, funding being linked to individual patients is a myth.

## Two conflicts

A conflict of worlds

The purpose of this aside at this point is not to stereotype, but to liberate you as reader to understand how two sets of understandable premises can lead to operational and philosophical conflict in CoC. The antagonists in this conflict are the doctors and the social workers.

World 1

'Classical' medicine presumes that health is freedom from disease. Medicine's objective is to restore health, and its purpose is therefore to do whatever will achieve cure. Hence, a doctor's primary duty is to focus on the pathology in hand, to achieve cure where possible, and, where not, to prolong life (death is failure in this value set). The patient's role is to allow necessary treatment to achieve medical health, and care is directed to 'look after the patient' whilst cure is being achieved.

In this world view, the best interest of a patient is self-evidently to trust the doctor since he or she possesses the knowledge of what is a person's medical best interest. Hence, logically, doctors must be paternalistic in deciding the best way of prolonging the patient's life and nurses ought to be 'maternalistic' in looking after the patient whilst the doctors solve the problem. This protective environment minimises risk and uncertainty, and leads ultimately to the assumption that a person can only be allowed to go home (and be restored to full autonomy) when they are healthy and therefore safe enough (i.e. when the doctor says so). This is of course waning as medicine embraces the principles of autonomy, although the default for the older generation of clinicians is paternalism and for patients is passivity.

### World 2

Conversely, social care and services operate from the premiss that health is independence and their purpose is to promote this. In this model, autonomy is centre stage and the risks and uncertainties that are part of an individual life are the substance of freedom. Hence, the respect of freedoms and choices in the place and nature of care have been givens for many years and patients have been seen as part of families and social networks within which illness and suffering must be interpreted. Nursing and the allied health professions have been considerably ahead of medicine in moving to the model of autonomy.

The result of this conflict is that doctors want people out of expensive beds when they have finished what they are able to do, but want them placed in environments that they consider to be safe, i.e. care homes, hospices or at worst at home with 24-hour care, and want it done now. Community services seldom have these capabilities on tap and, besides, the patient might not desire this model of care and informal carers may not be able or willing to provide it. Since informal carers will be charged with a caring role, their autonomy, which includes their right to refuse to offer care, also needs to be taken into account.

This, crudely, is an example in CoC of why there may be such tension in care. The solution is that both views need to move.

### A conflict of cost and cash flow

The second problem is more one of ideology than philosophy. There remains in the public and political mind the idea that we have a *National* Health Service and that it is integrated with social care. This is a myth. Modernisation, for entirely understandable political and macro-economic reasons, has led to the separation of provision into a series of interconnected but discrete businesses of which Foundation Trusts are exemplars.

This is fine in terms of fiscal accountability and the potential to reflect local need and relevance at a societal level, but may present real difficulties for individuals. The transfer of a patient from say a hospital to home or from home to a residential unit means that the saving in hospital bed days costs additional resources in community support that is not matched by a shift in funds. In terms of continuity of care, the impact on an individual's care package from unarticulated economic motives may limit options and damage communication.

---

**Box 14.2 Starting points in offering effective continuity of care**

- The principle of respect for autonomy is the central thread of continuity in care in which the patient knows his or her own best interest, even though it may be more uncertain and risky than paternalistic models.

- In circumstances of incapacity, valid Advance Decisions are legally binding; the legal authority of nominated representation (e.g. family) has changed and is virtually equivalent to the capable patient.

- The approach to care planning and continuity should be the same for institutional, community and home care.

- The philosophical conflict amongst the caring professions in offering consistency and continuity of care should now be historical.

- The new source of conflict is and will continue to be the problem of cash following the patient.

---

With the prominence of autonomy, you may well be asking now what duty one has in care other than to do what the patient demands. I come to this now.

## The duties of care

In this section we move from the view of the patient to the obligations and structures that deliver care: what we mean by a professional, how care is governed and how these inform teamwork. In 2002, an interesting volume of the *British Medical Journal* addressed various views of a good doctor.[6]

### *The notion of the professional*

Beauchamp and Childress[5,6,7] use a relatively restricted view of profession in considering health care that will open the discussion well. They identify distinct characteristics:

1. the provision of important services

2. personnel having had distinctive education, knowledge and training

3. rules of etiquette (courtesy etc.) and responsibilities to others in (for example) medicine, allied professions and the recipients of their services, and

4. the obligation to hold to general and specific moral norms of benefit, respect for the individual, etc.

These four criteria offer a cohesion, consistency and sense of identity for each profession, reassurance for society and *general* rules of engagement in one's work. Our respective governing bodies have codified these under the rubric Codes of Conduct or Duties of Care: some aspects have the force of statute, whereas others are explained or applied in specific situations as guidelines (e.g. withholding and withdrawing treatments). These form the foundations of effective practice, especially where there are potential conflicts in general and specific obligations, and in the mutuality and negotiation of distinct roles, responsibilities and authority that different professionals bring to effective seamlessness and continuity of care.

Being specific, the Royal College of Physicians has just completed a piece of work on medical professionalism in which it distinguishes the practice of medicine by the 'need for judgment in the face of extreme uncertainty' and defines medical professionalism as follows:

> Medicine is a vocation in which a doctor's knowledge, clinical skills and judgment are put in the service of protecting and restoring human well-being. This purpose is realised through a partnership between patient and doctor, one based on mutual respect, individual responsibility and appropriate accountability. In their day to day practice, doctors are committed to integrity, compassion, altruism, continuous improvement, excellence and working flexibly as part of dynamic clinical teams. These values, which underpin the science and practice of medicine, form the basis for a moral contract between the medical profession and society. Each party has a duty to work to strengthen the system of healthcare on which our collective human dignity depends.[8]

They then go on to make a requirement of doctors:

> We recommend that each doctor reflects on this definition and description of medical professionalism, recognising that he or she is a role model for doctors and other health care professionals. We further recommend that doctors assess their values, behaviours and relationships against this description, and that they take personal responsibility for ensuring that this aspirational standard of modern professionalism is met in their daily practice.

### Duties and obligations

Some general points

In truth, whilst many might wish it otherwise, there are very few absolute rules or responsibilities. For example, it is repugnant and indefensible to inflict pain on others for pleasure (this is an absolute in our society), but entirely necessary to 'inflict' the pain of surgery in order to evacuate a life-threatening extradural haematoma, or to set a displaced fracture. Consent one may say is mandatory, but that assumes this patient after his or her road traffic accident to be competent. We are under a general duty to benefit and to act in another's medical best interest, which trumps the requirement to allow the patient to succumb to haemorrhage or sepsis whilst we wait for them to permit the operations – that is of course unless there is a valid and specific advance statement or decision that foresaw the situation and refused the treatment. However, even then there may be grounds to resuscitate the patient under a general duty to act in presumption of life if the decision's scope or specificity is in question and there are other indications that the patient's view may have changed.

### Some areas of conflict or complexity

This leads us to see rights and freedoms such as autonomy, the consequent duties and general norms, as contingent or *prima-facie* obligations. That is to say: one's obligation is contingent upon other *potential or actual* duties being overridden, based on the facts, evaluations and defensible justifications for a given decision that are sufficient and 'good'.

This seems fairly straightforward, that is if there is a single view as to the patient's best interest. However, when we are dealing with cases where a patient is incapable, if several professionals are involved – especially from different disciplines – or where care is being given in different environments, then matters may become far more complicated. It should seem obvious in all situations that the process and basis for one's decision ought to be open and transparent, and the set course has been agreed by consensus. However, there are then other factors to consider:

1. to what degree is the patient capable of determining his or her care, or are there agreed advocates should he or she be incapable?

2. who has primary professional responsibility for the element of that patient's care under discussion and do they have sovereignty? Or

3. is this specific responsibility shared?

4. what other opinions and expertise should be brought reasonably to bear, and

5. how pressing or grave is the decision – on the one hand

limiting the time for consultation and on the other demanding the widest possible consensus?

I will return to this in the case of the extradural later (see cameo on Prof. Maelstrom, p. 260). First, we need to consider the codification of professionalism, namely the general matter of clinical governance and our duties to care.

## The governance of care

### *Professional duties*

The General Medical Council (GMC) and the Nursing and Midwifery Council (NMC) give good examples of the types of code that govern elements of the caring professions (see Table 14.1). They are different in important respects in that the NMC gives general instructions of what would define a good practitioner (one who is protective and supportive of client, community *and* colleague; competent, trustworthy, reputable and personally accountable), whereas the GMC seems more prescriptive and explicit about one's scope of competence, the need to collaborate with colleagues, the obligations of treatment and some assumptions about the doctor's ability to divine the best interest of another. You should note that, like the Royal College of Physicians' recommendations on professionalism, both, whilst concise, draw heavily on virtues such as trustworthiness, reputability, veracity, etc. One might claim to know what these mean, but they become strangely elusive to define when there is conflict in the air. These virtues seek to give an anatomy of what is good, but for our discussion it is the very issue of what is good, right or a best interest that will be in dispute if there is disagreement with a patient, his or her family or one's colleagues. For comparison, the latest version of the GMC's general guidance, which at the time of writing is currently out to consultation, appears in the second column of Table 14.1. The point is to show how it is moving more in the direction of general virtues rather than prescription.

Table 14.1 **DoH disclosure model for sharing confidential information**

| Core Guidance on Good Clinical Care (GMC, 2001)[9] | Core Guidance on Good Clinical Care (GMC Consultation, 2005)[10] | The NMC code of professional conduct: standards for conduct, performance and ethics ...[11] |
|---|---|---|
| Providing a good standard of practice and care | Patients must be able to trust doctors with their lives and health. To justify that trust you must: | As a registered nurse, midwife or specialist community public health nurse, you must |
| Good clinical care must include: | Respect human rights | ... have a duty of care to your patients and clients, who are entitled to receive safe and competent care |
| An adequate assessment; providing or arranging investigations or treatment ... taking suitable and prompt action, referring the patient to another practitioner, when indicated | Make the care of your patient your first concern | Act in such a way that justifies the trust and confidence the public have in you |
| In providing care you must: | Provide a good standard of practice and care | Uphold and enhance the good reputation of the professions |
| Be [clinically] competent ... recognis[ing] and work[ing] within the limits of your professional competence | Recognise and work within your professional competence | You are personally accountable for your practice. This means that you are answerable for your actions and omissions, regardless of advice or directions from another professional |
| Be willing to consult colleagues, keep[ing] [them] well informed when sharing care ... | Keep your professional knowledge and skills up to date | Protect and support the health of individual patients and clients |
| Provide the necessary care to alleviate pain and distress whether or not curative treatment is possible | Co-operate with colleagues | Protect and support the health of the wider community |

| | | |
|---|---|---|
| Keep clear, accurate, legible and contemporaneous patient records which report the relevant clinical findings, the decisions made, the information given to patients and any drugs or other treatment prescribed | Protect and promote the health of patients and the public | You must adhere to the laws of the country in which you are practising |
| Prescribe … only where you have adequate knowledge of the patient's health and medical needs, report[ing] adverse drug reactions … and co-operating with requests for information from organisations monitoring the public health | Act without delay if you have good reason to believe that you or a colleague is not fit to practise | |
| … not give or recommend … any investigation or treatment, which you know is not in their best interests, nor withhold appropriate treatments or referral | Make efficient use of the resources available to you | |
| Make efficient use of the resources available to you | Respect each patient's dignity and individuality | |
| If you have good reason to think that your ability to treat patients safely is seriously compromised … you should record your concerns and the steps you have taken to try to resolve them | Treat every patient politely and considerately | |

| |
|---|
| Respect patients' privacy and maintain confidentiality |
| Make sure your personal beliefs do not adversely affect patient care |
| Work with patients as partners in their care |
| Listen to patients |
| Give patients the information they want or need in a way they can understand |
| Respect patients' right to reach decisions with you about their treatment and care |
| Obtain informed consent where appropriate |
| Be honest and trustworthy |
| Never discriminate unfairly against patients or colleagues |
| Act with integrity |
| Be open with patients especially if something goes wrong |
| Never abuse your position as a doctor |
| Never act in ways which undermine public confidence in the medical profession |
| [Be] personally accountable |

*Source*: adapted from General Medical Council 2001,[9] General Medical Council 2006[10] and Nursing and Midwifery Council.[11]

**Teamworking: the moral contract for effective continuity of care**

We have reflected on the general issues that arise in continuity from professional and structural imperatives. The intended, practical solution is teamwork at various levels in health care. At a macro-level this is through National Service Frameworks for disease groups cascaded down through clinical networks to find expression in individual clinical cases with collaboration, joined up thinking and multidisciplinary teamwork. The central plank of CoC would seem, therefore, to be effective communication and teamwork. This is the basis of a moral contract between practitioners that matches with patients to complete a circle of mutuality.

*The elements*

Teams are groups of people set on a common goal with clear objectives, roles and rules of engagement – a good idea, except the simple definition hides a minefield of potential conflicts in values and assumptions. Success depends more on what is doable and the extent to which compromise is agreed than the ideals for which team members strive. This in turn falls to leadership. Most simply stated, there are four principal elements and four characteristics that bring both benefit and risk to effective teamwork (see Figure 14.1):

Four elements are at the arrow points in the diagram. *Power* and *influence* are essential in external relationships, but can be devastating internally if *any* individuals are disenfranchised or feel coerced. On the other hand, the compromises, time or processes for all to feel equal may paralyse decision making because any individual could veto any group decision. Hence, *expertise* and *influence* are necessary elements that place professionals in an appropriate (equitable) balance of relationship.

Taking the example of a patient with advanced neurodisability, the decision about pressure-relieving devices falls to the occupational therapist (OT) or whether to use a certain dressing are the domain of specialist and community nursing and not medicine; here respectively OT and nursing trump in decision making. On the other hand elements of diagnosis or therapeutics remain largely with medicine.

Figure 14.1 **Elements and characteristics of teamwork**

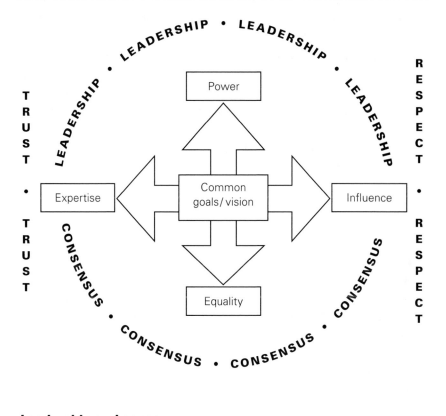

### Leadership and consensus

All teams need a leader. Mature teams, in which there is a high level of mutual trust and respect, when at their best, can operate without a discernible leader since the role will move around the group according to the domain under discussion. However, when an impasse is reached, the real leader and/or arbitrator will always emerge. Frequently the role is divided between a manager (someone who can get people to work together, administrate and complete tasks) and a leader (someone who can envision, motivate and excite). Traditionally in clinical teams, despite the fact that leadership and management are radically different skill sets, they have been rolled into one and the doctor is always assumed to be that person. However, this is disastrous when the individual does not have the skills, personality, character or motivation to lead or manage. This is no judgement on doctors who can't lead, but rather their emancipation. Teams need to be led by leaders: which discipline or speciality takes that role in any given team ought to be secondary.

The key to developing such a team is to build with an eye explicitly to the balances in personality and team roles as well as disciplines. I have, of course, presupposed that there is the resource and motivation in a service to develop effective teams and for there to be a routine element of team building and development recognised as an essential and legitimate part of the service delivery.

### Dealing with conflict and finding resolution

Risk analysis, professional duties and responsibilities lie at the centre of team processes and better the general utility of keeping as many in the team as happy as possible. In this respect, it is important that one understands very clearly and communicates to the team that their existence as a group is not an end in itself. Teams exist as a means to do 'the job' in the best and most effective way. Teams with strong bonds of commonality (and frequently social relationships that have flowed from their professional ones) are always at risk of seeing themselves as special, and the integrity of that team can subtly and insidiously become the real, subconscious goal of the group. All teams, but specialist ones in particular, are vulnerable to this.

Since ensuring effective service delivery is a function of clinical governance, the threat to this posed by dysfunctional teamworking should be seen as a governance issue for which a remedy needs to be found. The leader(s) must always keep this in mind when there is 'trouble at mill'. Readers are referred to the classical text for more explanation of teamworking.[12]

### The 'service(s)'

Whilst we all have duties and obligations as individual professionals, most practitioners are employed by organisations on behalf of whom they provide services to patients. In exchange, one may be indemnified. However, all professionals ultimately remain accountable to their professional governing bodies for their actions. In this respect, therefore, a clinician may find himself or herself at odds with his or her employer. The example of inadequate resources is given in the GMC Code. Discussion of this lies outside the scope of this chapter, but shows the clear link between one's employer, one's professional codes and the patient. Further, I would submit that the duties one has to patients and professionals must place one's employer last in the pecking order. It would also be a reasonable conclusion that one's relationship with others in configuring care ought to follow similar lines. This is central to today's practice as health and/or social care packages are assembled from proportionately complex relationships between organisations *per se* and through the relationships and responsibilities of individual professionals in individual cases. Where apparent conflicts of interest arise, discussion with colleagues and professional organisations are extremely useful as complex issues normally underlie such situations.

## Summary

Having laid some foundations for a general understanding of CoC, there are a handful of plumb lines that can be hung from the discussion so far:

1. there must be a presumption in favour of our patients' autonomy, and, wherever possible, this must be respected

2. there are attendant obligations to share information and seek opinions in decision making with
   a. the patient
   b. any advocates in situations of incapacity
   c. colleagues

3. communication and teamworking are the vehicle for effective CoC

4. there is an obligation to use resources wisely and effectively

5. for those working for organisations, there are attendant duties as an employee that will influence, but cannot outdo, one's duties to one's patient and profession.

## PARTICULAR APPLICATIONS

### Understanding and analysing areas of concern

So much for the principles and the general context of care. I now propose to use a handful of cases to cover areas where problems arise commonly and to demonstrate a way in which one can dismantle a case to expose underlying prejudices, inconsistencies or weaknesses in the analysis of a disagreement. In these disputes, some have clear rights and wrongs and solutions; others do not.

My primary purpose is not to prove what is right or wrong, but to demonstrate a practical and transparent way of coming to judgements that are defensible. I intentionally avoid recipes such as the four principles of autonomy and justice, beneficence and non-maleficence, or getting bogged down in meta-ethical theories. Instead, I wish to force a real engagement with practical reasoning that has a fighting chance of clarifying the basis of a dispute and through this to arrive at a strategy for resolving impediments to CoC.

This final ingredient (a practical reasoning process) is essential for successful navigation through the minefield of continuity as it helps practitioners see, when there are areas of conflict or dispute, where the differences between them lie. An effective method also allows teams to avoid conflict by using a coherent reasoning process from the word go. The following method is the one being developed and used by the multidisciplinary team at the Centre for Biomedical Ethics and Philosophy of Medicine at University College London (UCL) under the leadership of Janet Radcliffe Richards.

### *A method for practical reasoning*

In observing a pair of women engaged in a slanging match across their street, Dr Johnson once said that, 'it is impossible for neighbours in dispute to come to agreement, for they argue from different premises'. This is a truism since the basis of disputes, whilst often couched in claims about the facts of the matter, usually lie in the difference in antagonists' beliefs about what they take to be 'givens', that is to say their premises. And these are not based in facts about the way the world is, but in the values one holds about how the world ought to be. If an argument is unpicked to expose the ingredients of the dispute and define the basis of a disagreement, then there is the best chance of reaching a 'win:win' or of knowing at least what the true basis is for the disagreement. However, first there must be agreement as to what terms are to be used.

### Establishing a vocabulary

Two categories of question or information are involved in reaching a judgement. The first is the substance of the problem itself and other factual information that may be associated with or relevant to it and the second is the checks, balances, rights and wrongs, oughts and oughts not of the various options for action. No judgement is reached without the application, consciously or otherwise, of one or more of the category 2 – 'values' to category 1 – facts. In developing the approach to practical reasoning at UCL, we distinguish between these questions of 'fact' and questions of 'value' as the foundation from which to analyse the problem. However, we are not using the terms in their ordinary, vernacular sense.

### Questions of fact: what the issue is

These are matters concerning what the world is like and how it works, not how true or reliable are the data. For example, all questions of causes, effects and probability concern matters of fact as do statements of what someone may believe or hold to be good (the fact that he or she holds a view rather than the view itself). Because we decline these types of information as factual does not mean that one cannot have *beliefs, judgements, opinions, claims*, etc. about them. For example, if I claim that I can fly by flapping my arms I am making a claim of fact; if you say that this is nonsense, then you are making a judgement of fact. In other words, we are using fact to denote a *kind* of claim/belief/opinion etc., not to say how certain it may be.

### Questions of value: what matters in resolving the issue

Conversely, we are defining questions of value to be statements about what matters – what is good or bad, right or wrong, etc. These are the elements of our reasoning that move us in the direction of one set of actions over another. One's values may be moral in kind (about the way things ought to be), or they may be aesthetic (what looks good), selfish or emotive (what feels good), metaphysical or religious (referring to transcendent values) and so on. Again, one can make *claims* about these things, or have *beliefs*, *opinions* or views as to their truth etc.

### Borderlines

There are some pieces of information that cannot be categorised easily. For example, 'London is a large city' is clearly a factual judgement if you agree with the definition of large as, say, > 1,000,000 people, yet 'abstinence is the best form of contraception' is a value, but there feels to be a factual judgement behind it that turns on the word best – if one takes best to be most effective, then it is a judgement of fact, whereas sterilisation would be most effective if sex were considered to be essential. The law and professional standards are facts, since they are codifications of what society and the professions take to be good or right, although they are of course changing as they reflect the shifts in the value base of that society. In other words they are statements of the way things are, albeit based in what is expected that things ought to be.

### Bigger questions

The matter of whether there is any objective truth, and how we can know we have got there, is entirely separate from and peripheral to arbitrating between differing views of the facts of a case and judgements about what to do. Fortunately for us, the law and one's professional obligations and standards determine the parameters that we may for current purposes take as 'truths'.

### The process

### Establishing the facts

Since facts and values are different categories of information, the first task is to assign the data being used in an inquiry to one or other. It is best to begin by establishing the facts for two reasons:

   a. factual data are much less likely to be in dispute and if they are

   b. the basis for any dispute over facts will proceed from lack or mismatch in the information possessed by the antagonists.

Resolving the facts may lead to an immediate resolution of a problem. For example, if two consultants disagree over whether to offer some treatment, the fact of the patient's valid and applicable advance refusal resolves the dispute immediately; equally, discovering persuasive evidence about the disputed treatment is likely to abolish the divide between the clinicians.

*Listing the possible actions*
Oddly, it is often relatively easy to decide what one might do in a given situation without being aware of the value(s) that have been used in adjudicating between potential options, yet it is here that the source of dispute is usually spawned and where light can be shed.

*Discerning the values*
Having agreed and listed the facts and possible judgements/actions, the values are discerned by seeing which is necessary to get to each option. In this way, where one is deciding upon an action, this process allows one to test whether the value set being used is the right one. Where there is disagreement, one will expose the explicit or tacit value set and justification(s) that lie behind the differences of opinion. These may then be examined and subject in turn to acceptance or rejection until there is agreement, consensus or clarity as to the genuine basis of the disagreement. It is during this process that one finds two things: first, matters often claimed to be facts turn out to be tacit values; and, second, they can then be scrutinised against the law, standards, guidelines etc., as 'plumb lines' to bring resolution.

Finally, it is worth saying that reaching an agreement about an action doesn't mean one has automatically arrived there via the same values or that the values are good ones. For example, one surgeon may agree to a pulmonary lobectomy for bronchial carcinoma on a patient who resolutely continues to smoke because he or she is entitled to the operation, whilst another might feel that he or she doesn't deserve treatment, but agrees to the operation in order to give his or her registrar some practice.

This method of analysis will become clearer by working the following real but anonymised cases through which I will cover the principal areas in which dispute and conflicts occur. The first few are worked through in some detail, while the rest are left for your

Figure 14.2 **The process of practical reasoning**

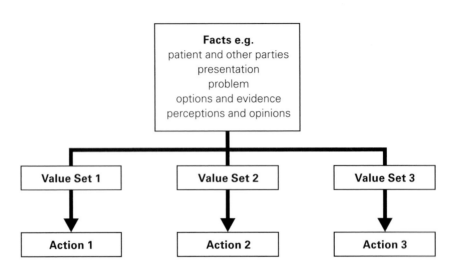

reflection. As one might imagine, disputes frequently originate from clashes of autonomy and perceived duties such as the professional's view of how a patient's interests are formulated.


**KEYS AREAS TO CONSIDER**

**Dealing with conflicts with colleagues**

***Clinical responsibility and delegating care***

Whether one likes it or not, power rather than patient interest still remains dangerously close to the heart of decision making. Furthermore, this is the worse for being entirely subconscious in many situations. This first example is the classical problem of the 'contraindication' and who decides on a treatment. A decision is made on the basis of what are stated to be facts when in truth the driver to the decision is an underlying value that assumes power to reside with the professional – or in some situations with the medical or 'senior' professional. See how effective practical reasoning is at exposing such motivations.

---

Cameo 1 **A dispute over medication**

---

Mr Smith is admitted to hospice for symptom control. He has grade IV heart failure, significant renal impairment previously exacerbated by NSAIDs and gout. He is on warfarin and a plethora of other drugs including thiazides. His joint pain is poorly controlled by opiates, which also make him drowsy and nauseated. These two things have all but abolished his limited mobility. He is very miserable and wanting to call it a day. Letters from the cardiologist and nephrologist to the GP say explicitly that NSAIDs are contraindicated despite reports that they control his arthralgia.

In discussion with Mr Smith, laying out the risks and benefits, a trial of diclofenac is agreed that abolishes his pain and restores mobility. However, his anticoagulation is difficult to control and there is a quantum reduction in his renal function.

Nevertheless, Mr Smith is much happier with this state of affairs as he is able to enjoy the garden.

In discussing the case with his GP, Dr Defer, and the decision to restart NSAIDs in particular, she expresses concern that this plan 'goes against the advice of the other two consultants'.

How should this be resolved and who takes the final decision?

The facts

a. The patient's symptoms are controlled but at the cost of renal function and there are drug interactions (*factual*).

b. The patient is informed of the issues, functional and happy; in other words, Mr Smith sees treatment to be in his best interest (*factual*).

c. The GP has reservations (*factual*).

d. Two other consultants say that the drugs are contraindicated. This may seem to be factual (the way things are); however, an indication is a value (the way it has been judged to be) stated as a fact; more precisely the *statement* of contraindication is a fact, but the *decision* that it is contraindicated is actually a value (much as the statement that a treatment is futile is treated by doctors as if it is a fact when it is actually a value).

What are the possible differences in the values and assumptions that lead the GP and the other consultants to think the NSAIDs should stop, when palliative care (and the patient) thinks that they should continue? We have a declared value (albeit stated as a fact) that doesn't really hold water. Some of the following offer more coherent possibilities:

Value set 1

   a. Consultants are the experts and the right action is the one recommended by the most of them (the proverbially responsible body).

   b. Because they are the experts, their view trumps both the GP and the patient.

   c. Generally this is tantamount to saying that the doctor knows what is in the best interest of the patient.

Value set 2

   a. 'Clinical health' is more important than global health, i.e. it is better to have normal renal function than to be free of pain.

   b. Prescribing what is safe is more important than what's effective.

There is therefore trouble here: 1a and b don't suggest teamwork, 1c violates autonomy and 2a and b exclude the patient altogether. The dispute is not in deciding who is wrong here (that makes winners and losers, a bad plan where consultants are concerned), but agreeing the purpose and objectives of the treatment.

Defining questions

These comments may seem over-critical. However, the following questions will soon expose the first-order value(s) that are driving the dispute:

   a. What is the primary purpose of treatment in this case?

   b. Is a complication always a reason to stop treatment? If so, then

   c. Who determines that something is a complication of a *symptomatic* treatment, the doctor or the patient?

   d. Where does the patient stand in relation to requests for treatment; is it he or she who determines what is an unacceptable risk?

Means to resolution

One thing is clear in this analysis, the GP feels that Mr Smith ought not to judge for himself. This flies in the face of both the law and standards. The issue cannot be the different opinions of the consultants if we establish the objective of treatment to be symptom control and the patient to consider the risks to be worth it.

The problem was solved when the GP saw Mr Smith to confirm that he was fully informed and prioritised mobility and analgesia above his longevity. The hospital consultants were of course quite happy with this decision once Mr Smith's wishes and priorities were known and felt no need to take centre stage in future decisions.

The implications for continuity

People are designed to live at home, so the lynchpin of continuity in care is general practice. The point of this case is to show that the GP is perfectly entitled to trump the views of any consultant in deciding on the best treatment of his or her patients and that, for effective continuity of care, treatments may need to be the subject of discussion rather than just instruction.

## Deciding between active and palliative management

This is a much more complex problem framing itself as a simple question of active or palliative care. It highlights the problem of incapacity and its state of permanence, the change in the authority of family in decision making and how decisions that appear simple and stark are nothing of the sort. Application of the new Mental Capacity Act clarifies this to some extent.

In this case, two consultants are also going head to head: guidelines and the literature are effectively silent when it comes to who trumps who over treatment except to say that colleagues should respect one another's opinions and base their practice as far as possible on evidence.

The initial facts

1. This is an acute clinical problem, which on face value needs action within hours.

2. There is a judgement on the facts, namely the reversibility of the problem.

---

Cameo 2  **Advance statements, incapacity and best interests**

---

Prof. Maelstrom is a retired philosopher with early Alzheimer's disease. She lives alone, is fiercely independent, but muddled at times and reluctantly has agreed to some social care. She is able to get out and is known in her area such that a watchful eye is kept upon her. One morning, she is knocked over by a motorcyclist and is admitted to casualty with a skull fracture and becomes unconscious. A CT scan shows an extradural haematoma. The casualty consultant has alerted the neurosurgeons and plans are being made for transfer when the professor's brother and sister arrive.

It transpires that she has always been adamant that should she begin 'losing her mind' that the quicker she died the better. None of this is in writing, but she is a member of the Voluntary Euthanasia Society. The casualty consultant now revises her view as to the wisdom of referring for surgery. However, the neurosurgeon is horrified and says that leaving her is at best negligence and at worst euthanasia by omission.

---

Value set 1

There appears to be no question as to the value set of both the neuro-surgeon and the A & E consultant at the initial presentation: both are operating on a presumption in favour of life and an assumption, in the absence of information to the contrary, that the professor is temporarily incapable and treatment should return her to her former health.

Initial judgement and action

This then leads to the first action, referral for evacuation. Both consultants are in agreement and that seems to be the end of the matter.

Further information

However, circumstances change dramatically as new facts emerge:

3. Only later does it become apparent that the professor also has background chronic progressive disease.

4. Statements of fact are also made about quality of life by the family.

5. The surgeon is presenting the dispute as a double whammy: one of fact (stated) and of value (implied).

    a. Negligence is a factual claim: the right treatment is … and you have failed to give it.

b. The second factual claim is that non-treatment is euthanasia. It is wrong, but the implied value is that the A & E consultant doesn't value life.

This is an aggressive and highly judgemental interaction.

It is only with the new information suggesting that the professor may have refused this treatment plan that a chasm begins to open between them.

### Value set 2

The A & E consultant's presumption is contingent upon the 'type', quality or indeed acceptability of that life to its owner, or that presumption in favour of life doesn't mean treatment at all costs – i.e. the right to life does not necessarily mean the right to be kept alive at all costs, but the right not to be killed.

The neurosurgeon's position seems to be an absolute presumption in favour of life.

### Defining questions

There are a number of factual assumptions (i.e. judgements and claims). These need clarification and may help the surgeon on the one hand to engage the individual in this case and possibly the A & E consultant to reverse her decision. The important ones are listed on Table 14.2.

Table 14.2 **Facts for and against surgery**

| Possible additional facts in favour of surgery | Possible additional facts against surgery |
| --- | --- |
| What probability is there that non-treatment will lead to rapid deterioration and death? Or stated another way: | Of course, evacuation may only be partially successful in restoring Prof. Maelstrom, who may stabilise at a much lower functional level and be 'worse off than dead' |
| With no action, how likely is it that Prof. Maelstrom could stabilise and be 'worse off than dead' according to opinions from the family | What is the certainty of evidence that evacuation will lead to complete recovery? |
| | What is the likelihood of anaesthetic risk with possible cognitive deterioration? And: |
| | How certain is it that rehabilitation will be successful? |

### Means to resolution

The continuity issue here is substantial since Prof. Maelstrom is currently known to health and social services. A number of professionals also know the case and doubtless have opinions about the professor's views.

Standards and professionalism dictate our obligations in decision making. In this case, on the one hand we are to begin from a presumption in favour of life, but on the other we need very good reasons to overrule autonomy. In this case the A & E consultant appears to be in the right. Whilst Advance Refusals need not be written, the Mental Capacity Act is clear that, where such refusals are likely to lead to an earlier death, then they must be written.[5] In all circumstances, they must be specific, e.g. in covering acute or unexpected events and their scope, in covering reversibility, and uncertainty of outcome must be sufficient for the circumstance to be considered valid.

### Implications for continuity

Depending on the time of day and urgency, the GP's opinion as the person responsible for continuing the professor's management seems most important and should be sought as a matter of urgency. However, it is essential to note relevant elements of the Mental Capacity Act. It is clear about advanced decisions specificity, scope and validity and in the case of potentially 'fatal' refusals, these need to be written. Second, section 4 gives clear criteria for assessing best interest taking into account *inter alia* (s.4c) iv:

a. '... the patient's past and present wishes and feelings (and in particular any relevant written statement made by the patient whilst he had capacity);

b. The beliefs and values that would be likely to influence the patient's decision if he had capacity;

c. any other factors the patient would consider if able to do so.

[also] ... Take account, if practicable, of views as to what would be in P's best interests of: anyone named by P as someone to be consulted; anyone engaged in caring for P or interested in his welfare; any holder of a legal power of Attorney; any Court Appointed Deputy.'

Members of the family may have enduring power of attorney that extends to decisions over care. It is important to be familiar with this new development in the law.

To summarise this case, either course of action is defensible. On the matter of who trumps whom, it would seem reasonable that it is the consultant under whose care the patient finds himself or herself. In this case, it is the A & E consultant. Whatever the decision, the respective consultants will have to be prepared to defend themselves.

## Continuity of care where patients exercise their freedom to 'refuse'

General points

One of the principal drivers for caring professionals is that they are there to do good and to improve their patients'/clients' wellbeing through treatments or care. This is the whole idea of a patient's best interest from that professional's perspective. However, as we are beginning to perceive and apply the ramifications of the principle of autonomy (that the capable patient is the one who knows and has custody of his or her best interest), a continuing pressure will come on clinicians to navigate through increasingly complex cases where patients need not be consistent, rational or predictable. The task is to define the respective responsibilities and limits that apply to this principle in action.

Just to be clear, it is worth reiterating the scope of refusal before we look at a handful of cases.

1. Provided that an individual is capable – i.e. able to understand, evaluate and judge information – then their statement of their best interest is absolute, regardless of whether it is 'eccentric or unwise'.

2. The temptation may be overwhelming to assume that, because a patient comes to what one considers to be a stupid or wrong decision, they are incapable. This must be resisted as this freedom to expose oneself to harm or even fatality is a matter of law.[4]

This next example (cameo 3) shows how a clinician seems to think that he or she can overrule her patient and colleague on no other grounds than that the patient has refused.

---

Cameo 3 **Deciding what's best**

Mrs Snyder is 60, and lives alone. She has had chronic myeloid leukemia (CML) for several years. One day she calls her GP, Dr Black, saying she is dizzy, in pain and has been vomiting. She is out, so Dr White, one of Dr Black's partners, makes the house call.

He finds she has had a myocardial infarction, and advises immediate admission to hospital. Mrs Snyder flatly refuses, and points to a sheet of paper propped behind the telephone, which is a valid and specific living will declaring that she does not want to be admitted to hospital under any circumstances.

Dr White reluctantly agrees to treat her as well as he can at home. He returns to the practice to find that Dr Black has returned. She says that Mrs Snyder's refusal is absurd, and that she will get her to hospital. Dr Black does this by saying that she really does need to go to A&E for tests, but that she won't need to stay. On that basis Mrs Snyder agrees to go to the hospital where – as her GP expects – she is immediately admitted to the coronary unit.

---

The facts

1. A capable patient refuses the suggested management for a cardiac problem.

2. A valid advanced statement supports the notion that this refusal is a reflection of an enduring view by Mrs Snyder.

3. Her view is respected by one GP and overruled by the second who has also coerced the patient by deception.

Value set 1

*Dr Black*: the only explanation for her actions that bears any resemblance to a defensible position is that she considers admission to be in Mrs Snyder's best interest and this is indeed what she claimed.

*Dr White* respects Mrs Snyder's valid refusal, whilst not considering it her best interest: Note that whilst Dr White's opinion as to Mrs Snyder's best interest is the same, his action distinguishes a different set of values.

Since 'best interests' cannot be the root of Dr Black's action (quite simply because Mrs Snyder is capable) and Dr Black's use of 'absurd' indicates that she believes that there is either a correct course of action (i.e. rational) or a right course of action (i.e. moral). Neither position is justifiable according to either the law or professional standards (see Table 14.1 on p. 245). So what are the possible values behind Dr Black's actions?

Other possible value sets

1.  It's wrong for a patient to prevent a curative treatment (*value*).

2.  I am the doctor, so I know my patients' best interests (*a value stated as a fact*).

3.  The correct management is admission (*factual claim*), so I must not be prevented from doing the correct thing (*value*). Why?

4.  Because judgement is nothing more than doing the correct thing (*factual claim about a value*), or

5.  Being prevented from doing the correct thing exposes doctors to charges of negligence (*factual claim*), i.e. a doctor's best interest trumps a patient's best interest (*value*).

Means to resolution

The continuity issues here are rather serious. I suggest that Dr White cannot let this matter pass unchallenged because the actions of Dr Black show that she considers his actions to have been either wrong or unprofessional. For trust to be maintained in the practice, this has to be resolved. Equally, I assume that Dr White holds the patient's freedoms in high regard and would find lying or coercion to be a form of battery that falls short of physical violation but equal in its moral unacceptability.

A direct conversation between the GPs found no common ground, so the matter was resolved by using an external expert to analyse the case as a study example of refusals in the practice's educational meeting. Once Dr Black realised that her underlying values could not have been to act in her patient's best interest, and that she had in fact breached professional standards and could have been liable in law, she was horrified and very repentant.

### Balance of duties of care with autonomy or best interests in the vulnerable patient

---

Cameo 4 **Care packages that cannot be sustained**

---

Monica Brand has a 2-year history of motor neurone disease and, whilst she is still able to talk, swallow and operate a TV remote control, she is otherwise entirely dependent.

She has professional carers during the day and a district nurse visits her day and night. Her partner is unable to be involved consistently in her care as he has a peripatetic job that takes him away from home several days and nights a week.

Monica has a full-thickness sacral pressure sore with recurrent infection and bleeding. She refuses procedures and pressure care to minimise this, preferring to stay in her chair all day. She is now symptomatic from anaemia, but refuses admission for transfusion.

Managing these packages has been difficult: on average, care agencies have lasted about six months as Monica has systematically complained about and eventually refused entry to individual carers in each team. She has also run into difficulties with respite admissions to two local hospices and acute admissions to the three local acute hospitals. She has complained about all formally.

The fourth care agency has run out of carers acceptable to Monica. Her professional care is due to terminate in one week and no other agencies are available or willing to step in. Monica is aware of this but refuses admission anywhere, even in the short term.

The meeting comprises commissioners, community nursing, palliative care and care agencies. The preoccupation is with ensuring Monica's welfare and how she can be persuaded to change her mind.

---

It may seem inconceivable to consider leaving a patient at home unattended who is in need of constant care. Consider this case from Mrs Brand's position, remembering that she is capable and therefore free to be irrational or unwise and see if it is possible to come out with another action that does not violate her autonomy.

### The implications for continuity

The outcome was that the community staff and final care agency crumbled and, despite considerable personal morbidity, they continued to offer care for this patient until she died. However, the outcome was a substantial tightening of referral policy, eligibility and the contract between patients and carers. Some would say that other patients following her care have suffered as a result of her actions.

## Dealing with uncertainty

Cameo 5 **A difference of opinion over emergency drugs**

It was a Friday morning and Audrey Gray's clinical condition was deteriorating. She had adenocarcinomatosis; she was nauseous and having trouble keeping medication down. Her community palliative care clinical nurse specialist (CNS) assessed her after a request from the family and judged that she was beginning to enter the dying process. Her pain was well controlled on MST 60 mg bd, but she was an anxious lady and fearful of having to leave her home. The CNS rang the GP and asked for emergency supplies of parenteral drugs including diamorphine and midazolam for the house. He visited and things had settled. He left a 5 mg vial of diamorphine and some cyclizine.

On checking the situation that afternoon, the CNS, who was very experienced and knew the patient well, was concerned that this was inadequate given the uncertainty of her condition and rang the GP back for a discussion. It went badly and she spoke to the hospice consultant, who agreed that, whilst not having seen Mrs Gray, should she deteriorate and need injectables, one dose of diamorphine was insufficient. He rang the GP again.

The conversation went equally badly, but for different reasons. What do you think they might have been and why?

The patient was fine over the weekend. On the Monday morning, there is a letter copied to you that the GP has sent to the PCT head pharmacist.

Try putting together your own analysis of this case. Here was my approach:

The issue was not whether Mrs Gray was in need of a syringe driver there and then, or indeed whether she would need one at all, but the continuity of her care: who was to be responsible for her clinical care that weekend? The community nursing service only covers to 11 p.m. and, whilst this palliative care team offers an on-call service, the staff do not carry drugs. Since the GP had not made the resources available for the palliative care team to be able to discharge their on-call responsibility (i.e. adequate drug supplies were not in the house to cover reasonable eventualities), who should the family contact in an emergency?

Was the GP himself on call? If so, then no problem: he had made a clinical judgement; there was provision in the house for the community nurses to give an injection to cover an emergency during the day and the doctor had four hours to reassess. The consultant checked his assumption that a night call would go straight through to the GP.

Was another GP in the practice or the deputising service on? If so who would inform them of the situation? Was the GP willing to take responsibility if Mrs Gray's care was deficient over that weekend?

Mrs Gray had no drugs that weekend and was fine. The conversation was subject to a letter of complaint from the GP to the PCT's chief pharmacist on the Monday morning complaining about the events of Friday because they undermined his authority and autonomy as GP. It was not said outright, but the tone of the letter implies that the plan was to over-analgese and over-sedate the patient. It emerges that this GP has a history of referring symptomatic patients late to specialist services. Following a response from the consultant, the matter was handled by the practice manager and senior partner, and a protocol was established for emergency drug provision in the home.

## Dealing with conflicts of interest

### Confidentiality

Continuity by definition requires information to be shared. Understanding confidentiality is therefore of the utmost importance in this discussion.

Confidentiality means 'with faith or trust' and is a cornerstone of any viable clinical relationship. Without trust there is no reliable reference point for a therapeutic relationship. However, there are circumstances where problems arise between professionals as a result of strictures applied by the patient. Without sounding like a cracked record, confidentiality is another expression of the principle of autonomy and, again, problems only really arise when patients exercise their right to privacy. To be blunt, any information relating to a patient belongs to them – one doesn't give, or even lend, a friend's car to someone without seeking permission – and the same applies to personal information. However, it is more than that: one's privacy, in the radical individualistic framework of the West, at least, is an element of defining our individuality and uniqueness. As with treatment refusals, when sharing information it is necessary to promote what we believe to be the patient's interest; the principles we have explored above apply.

However, information is different in two ways: first, it may have direct impact on the interests of others; and, second, it is also factual according to our definition. In relation to others, we have duties that relate to public interest of one sort or another. In relation to the information itself, because it is factual, discussing and determining the way in which we handle it becomes simpler than when values are involved centre stage. Nevertheless, one must recognise that information that is entirely innocuous to one person may be a very private matter to another. It is therefore generally unacceptable to disclose without seeking permission, even if we are under obligation to disclose under the circumstances below.

### General guidance

*Presumption in favour of confidentiality*
First, let's set the basic parameters. Since one *prima-facie* human right is privacy,[13] there must be a presumption in favour of confidentiality. This means in straightforward terms that one is obliged always to gain permission before discussing a patient's details with *anyone*; of course, this is subject to some common sense in that there is assumed and tacit consent in coming into the surgery or with out-patients that the administrators, nurses, doctors and other clinicians have access to the information necessary and sufficient to fulfil their duty of care. The point is that simply being an employee is not *carte blanche* for anyone in a surgery to have access to all information. Disclosure is only justified by a professional need to know. Confidentiality is sufficiently important in health care to merit a dedicated publication on the Code of Practice from the Department of Health (DoH).[14]

*The need to know*
The starting point in deciding on disclosure is the necessity to fulfil one's duty of care. Clearly, a receptionist doesn't need a patient's sexual history to identify them, but does need, say, a date of birth or address. However, there is still the default that a patient can refuse to disclose any information. That may restrict the services he or she

can access, but the freedom is his or hers to choose.

The most obvious need to know is when there is a substantial risk to another as expressed below in the DoH Code of Practice.

> Disclosure of personal information without consent may be justified where failure to do so may expose the patient or others to risk of death or serious harm. Where third parties are exposed to a risk so serious that it outweighs the patient's privacy interest, you should seek consent to disclosure where practicable. If it is not practicable, you should disclose information promptly to an appropriate person or authority. You should generally inform the patient before disclosing the information [para: 36].[14]

Fortunately further on in the Code of Practice, more detail is given as to how one defines the 'Need to Know' [para. 38]. Table 14.3 gives the questions one should ask in deciding whether to disclose. The algorithm from Annex B gives what the DoH considers the correct process.

Table 14.3 **Determining disclosure**

| | |
|---|---|
| *If the purpose served by disclosing is not healthcare or another medical purpose, what is the basis in administrative law for disclosing?* | Public sector bodies should only do the things that they have been set up to do. Whilst medical purposes are permitted, disclosures to other agencies for other purposes may not be |
| *Is disclosure either a statutory requirement or required by order of a court?* | Although disclosure should be limited to that required and there may be scope to ask the court to amend an order, at the end of the day any disclosure that has either a statutory requirement or court order must be complied with |
| *Is the disclosure needed to support the provision of healthcare or to assure the quality of that care?* | Patients understand that some information about them must be shared in order to provide them with care and treatment, and clinical audit, conducted locally within organisations is also essential if the quality of care is to be sustained and improved. Efforts must be made to provide information, check understanding, reconcile concerns and honour objections. Where this is done there is no need to seek explicit patient consent each time information is shared[4] |

| | |
|---|---|
| *If not healthcare, is the disclosure to support a broader medical purpose?* | Preventative medicine, medical research, health service management, epidemiology etc. are all medical purposes as defined in law. Whilst these uses of information may not be understood by the majority of patients, they are still important and legitimate pursuits for health service staff and organisations. However, the explicit consent of patients must be sought for information about them to be disclosed for these purposes in an identifiable form unless disclosure is exceptionally justified in the public interest or has temporary support in law under section 60 of the Health & Social Care Act 2001. |
| *Is the use of identifiable and confidential patient information justified by the purpose?* | Where the purpose served is not to provide healthcare to a patient and is not to satisfy a legal obligation, disclosure should be tested for appropriateness and necessity, with the aim of minimising the identifiable information disclosed and anonymising information wherever practicable. |
| *Have appropriate steps been taken to inform patients about proposed disclosures?* | There is a specific legal obligation to inform patients in general terms, who sees information about them and for what purposes. Where the purpose of providing information is also to seek consent, more detail may be necessary and patients need to be made aware of their rights and how to exert them. See Annex A2 for more detail. |
| *Is the explicit consent of a patient needed for a disclosure to be lawful?* | Unless disclosure of identifiable patient information is required by law or the courts, is for a healthcare purpose, can be justified as sufficiently in the public interest to warrant breach of confidence, or is supported by section 60 of the Health & Social Care Act 2001, explicit consent is required. |
| *NB: any 'other' organisational forms of audit, i.e. across organisations and nationally, require explicit consent* | |

*Source*: DoH,[14] p. 15.

*Agreeing rules of engagement*

An area that presents particular challenges to teamworking is when colleagues are denied information. To what degree do colleagues have a need to know and what values might apply? Here are two cases: the first motivated by power, the second by fear.

---

Cameo 6 **Confidentiality without clear purpose**

A colleague whose partner was dying asked to use our social worker for counselling and support. He held her to complete confidentiality and spent the subsequent weeks criticising and undermining the team's care. It was very destructive of relationships within the team as the social worker was inexperienced, unsure of the validity of the criticisms and feeling unable to check or resolve the problem. Matters eventually came to a head.

---

I well recall a case many years ago in which we used practical reasoning to decide on our course of action.

The facts
1. The carer (C) had asked for counselling and support.

2. He spoke of a number of areas of the patient's (P) care that were unsatisfactory in his opinion.

Value set 1
1. Counselling ought to help C to cope and to that end

2. It should identify areas of difficulty where remedy is possible and

3. Offer coping strategies for areas that are practically insoluble.

Interim judgement and actions
C presented a variety of remediable complaints, suggesting that he saw this as the place to air them and the social worker asked for the opportunity to address them discreetly with the team.

Discriminating facts
3. C refused to allow the social worker to disclose problems for them to be engaged, saying that

4. Whilst the complaints recurred at each counselling session, C said he didn't want to make a fuss.

Figure 14.3 **Disclosure model**

**B1: Disclosure Model[11]– where it is proposed to share confidential information in order to provide healthcare**

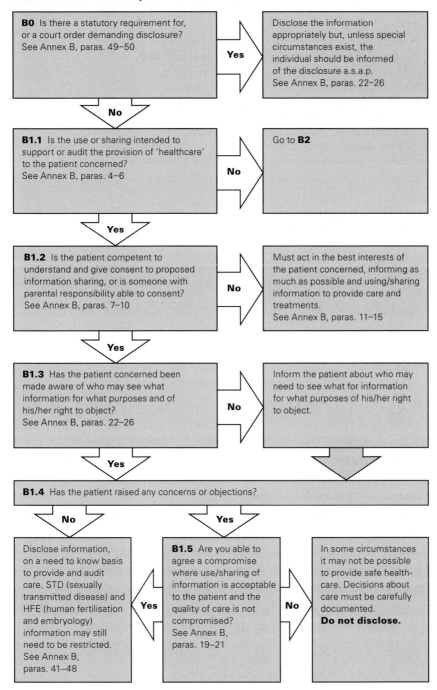

**B0** Is there a statutory requirement for, or a court order demanding disclosure? See Annex B, paras. 49–50

→ **Yes** → Disclose the information appropriately but, unless special circumstances exist, the individual should be informed of the disclosure a.s.a.p. See Annex B, paras. 22–26

↓ **No**

**B1.1** Is the use or sharing intended to support or audit the provision of 'healthcare' to the patient concerned? See Annex B, paras. 4–6

→ **No** → Go to **B2**

↓ **Yes**

**B1.2** Is the patient competent to understand and give consent to proposed information sharing, or is someone with parental responsibility able to consent? See Annex B, paras. 7–10

→ **No** → Must act in the best interests of the patient concerned, informing as much as possible and using/sharing information to provide care and treatments. See Annex B, paras. 11–15

↓ **Yes**

**B1.3** Has the patient concerned been made aware of who may see what information for what purposes and of his/her right to object? See Annex B, paras. 22–26

→ **No** → Inform the patient about who may need to see what for information for what purposes of his/her right to object.

↓ **Yes**

**B1.4** Has the patient raised any concerns or objections?

↙ **No**

Disclose information, on a need to know basis to provide and audit care. STD (sexually transmitted disease) and HFE (human fertilisation and embryology) information may still need to be restricted. See Annex B, paras. 41–48

↓ **Yes**

**B1.5** Are you able to agree a compromise where use/sharing of information is acceptable to the patient and the quality of care is not compromised? See Annex B, paras. 19–21

← **Yes**

→ **No** → In some circumstances it may not be possible to provide safe health-care. Decisions about care must be carefully documented. **Do not disclose.**

*Note*: B2 is 'Disclosure Model' – where the purpose isn't health care but it is a medical purpose as defined in the legislation – another suggested algorithm. *Source*: DoH.[14]

5. Hence, the complaints were either in sufficient or another motive underlay them (both judgements on the facts).

6. C's claims were damaging the effectiveness of the service in delivering care, not just to this patient, but to others through difficulties between the social worker and the rest of the team.

### Means to resolution

There are two sets of duties to care: one to the patient (P) and the other to the carer (C). Are there any justifications for disclosure and to what degree may P trump C?

1. The disclosure is to other health carers and so the information remains contained in a group with statutory obligations of confidentiality.

2. The information relates to the delivery of care to P.

3. The continuity of care was being compromised by C.
   a. Directly in that there may actually be justifiable criticisms of the care that needed to be addressed, and
   b. Indirectly by undermining the team's functionality and attempt to deliver care.

4. The team's primary duty of care was to P. C's entitlement to support was as part of that care. Otherwise, his support would have come from elsewhere.

There seems to be sufficient justification to disclose to the team. However, to what extent?

5. The social worker arguably is also being compromised in her ability to provide support in that C is frustrating any attempt to address his putative concerns. This is his freedom, but limits his benefit.

6. However, it does not mean that everything said to the social worker should be available to all. Personal matters remain just that.

The social worker disclosed her difficulties to her supervisor, who spoke to the team leader. There was a general discussion about the justifiable scope of confidentiality and the duty of care to the patient. Some of the criticisms were justifiable and were addressed discreetly. The others were largely a function of C's own issues and judged not to indicate a problem within the team. Since C did not want to take things further and make a formal complaint the issues were allowed to pass.

### The implications for continuity

The upshot of this for the team was a clear policy with families that discussion with any member of the team was the same as discussion with the team itself. Any wish for tighter confidentiality would then be open to discussion explicitly to minimise the risk of potential fragmentation.

To conclude, consider the following case where the continuity issue is not simply the need of the patient, but of her dependents. This is the key to the case. The challenge then is to offer the patient the facts rather than being driven by her perceptions and fears.

Consider here how you would construct the arguments and justifications for disclosure or confidentiality.

We elected to speak very frankly to the patient about the needs of the children and their entitlements as British citizens. We also said

---

**Cameo 5  Confidentiality, disclosure and conflicting interests**

Mrs Umbala has an operably curable thyroid cancer and is refusing surgery. She has said to her oncology CNS that this is because she cannot arrange care for her two small children whilst in hospital. There is considerable concern that in delaying treatment the tumour will be inoperable. Social services are already involved in the case following some problems with the children at school.

Mrs Umbala is estranged from their father. The oncology CNS knows that she has very little in the way of social support, although she is adamant with the social worker that she can cope and has family help. She is clearly unwell and defensive when she is asked about her health. The social worker is keen to be of assistance and knows that Mrs Umbala is having hospital treatment, but she has forbidden the CNS to speak to the social worker about her illness. This has led to a lot of tension between the two professionals. However, it emerges in discussion that, whilst Mrs Umbala has been in this country for several years and both children were born in England, she entered with a tourist visa and has no legal right to be here. This explains her anxiety about social service involvement and child care. She is terrified that the children will be taken into care and she will be deported. She may also be worrying that she will have to pay for hospital care.

that we would have to inform the social worker of the situation as a duty to them as minors. She agreed and once she was reassured that they would not be taken from her, Mrs Umbala had her surgery free of charge. She is now complaining about what she sees to be inadequate accommodation for her and her children, and is proving a handful.

## CONCLUSION

The purpose of this chapter has been to consider why we ought to foster continuity of care. We have tested the grounds for this: our duties and responsibilities as professionals that flow from treating patients as ends and not means, and seeking clinically and economically effective care. We have also considered ways to make this real through teamworking and considering some examples in areas where difficulties commonly arise. However, the purpose of this has been to offer a way in which to use practical reasoning to reach solutions rather than to be a digest of recipes to solve clinical conflict.

## REFERENCES

1. Harris J. *Assisted Dying for the Terminally Ill Bill.* 86-I, 20, para. 41. London: The Stationery Office, 2005.

2. *Re B (Adult: Refusal of Medical Treatment)* 2. re B. 449 [2]. 2002. All England Reports.

3. Phillips M, Waller L J and Wall L J. *Burke, R (on the application of) v General Medical Council & Ors.* EWCA Civ 1003 (28 July 2005). Available from: www.bailii.org/ew/cases/EWCA/Civ/2005/1003.html [accessed March 2007].

4. Department of Constitutional Affairs. *The Mental Capacity Act.* London: Department of Constitutional Affairs, 2005.

5. National Council for Palliative Care. *Guidance on the Mental Capacity Act.* London: National Council for Palliative Care, 2005.

6. Various. What's a good doctor and how do you make one? *British Medical Journal* 2002; **325**: 667–724.

7. Beauchamp T L and Childress J F. *Principles of Biomedical Ethics.* New York: Oxford University Press, 2001.

8. Royal College of Physicians of London. *Doctors in Society. Medical professionalism in a changing world.* London: RCP, 2005.

9. General Medical Council. *Good Medical Practice.* 3rd edition. London: General Medical Council, 2001.

10. General Medical Council. *Good Medical Practice.* London: General Medical Council, 2006.

11. Nursing and Midwifery Council. *The NMC Code of Professional Conduct: Standards for conduct, performance and ethics.* London: Nursing and Midwifery Council, 2004.

12. Speck P (ed.). *Teamwork in Palliative Care: Fulfilling or frustrating.* Oxford: Oxford University Press, 2006.

13. United Nations. Universal Declaration of Human Rights. 1948. Available at: http://webworld.unesco.org/water/wwap/pccp/cd/pdf/educational_tools/course_modules/reference_documents/internationalregionconventions/universal declarationhumanrights.pdf [accessed March 2007].

14. Department of Health. Confidentiality NHS Code of Practice, 2003. Available from: www.dh.gov.uk/assetRoot/04/06/92/54/04069254.pdf [accessed March 2007].

CHAPTER | 15

# Postscript

Palliative care continuity in the new NHS

*Dan Munday, Cathy Shipman and Scott A. Murray*

---

## Palliative care and continuity – definitions and scope

Almost 40 years ago, Dame Cicely Saunders established St Christopher's Hospice in Southeast London. Since that time palliative care has developed exponentially. It has expanded globally as hospices have emerged throughout the economically developed and developing world; a new speciality of palliative care has been established, with branches in medicine, nursing, allied professions, social and spiritual care. In addition, it has extended into hospitals and community care, and become part of mainstream healthcare provision. It is now seen increasingly as relevant and necessary for end-of-life care for any progressive illness, with calls for palliative care to be provided for patients with cancer from the moment of diagnosis.

### What is palliative care?

Although the concept of palliative care has been defined and redefined, its scope has increased so widely it is pertinent to ask 'What actually is palliative care?' and 'How does it differ from a caring holistic approach of healthcare professionals to all of their patients?' It seems that palliative care is commonly defined in two different ways. First, it is defined as a system for control of symptoms for patients with advanced, incurable illnesses requiring specialist knowledge and skills, with many different disciplines working in an integrated fashion, i.e. medicine, nursing, rehabilitation therapies, counselling, spiritual care, etc. Second, palliative care is defined as a 'philosophy', where the focus is on supportive care that includes a holistic, patient-centred approach with good communication and teamworking as central. Many aspects of this second definition are closely related to traditional primary care, which also strives to offer patient-centred holistic care using a teamwork approach. This type of care should arguably be extended not just to those at the end of life, but those at the beginning and in the middle also, since this form of care is needed by any patient and his or her family facing a significant illness, whether acute or chronic, physical or psychological, clearly diagnosed or with an elusive diagnosis (as commonly encountered in primary care).

Palliative care's substantive nature is also often unclear. It is commonly proposed, for instance in National Service Frameworks, that palliative care is an important aspect of care for patients with advanced cardiac, neurological and renal disorders, and also patients with dementia. However, it is rarely explicit exactly what such palliative care should involve or who should be responsible for its delivery. How should it operate in conjunction with other aspects of care for such patients? Should specialist management be provided by specialists in palliative care or specialists for the condition for which palliative care is required? Should non-cancer patients be admitted to hospices and do these institutions have staff with the skills and equipment to manage them safely and effectively? It is likely that specific models will need to be developed to meet the needs of people with each condition and different models may well be required for the same condition but in different geographical and organisational contexts. Answers to these questions are unlikely to be forthcoming without extensive research, requiring adequate funding and novel research methods to enable a clear understanding of the issues and possible solutions to emerge.

### What is continuity of care?

This book has focused on the provision of continuity of care for the palliative care patient. Whilst the definition and scope of palliative care is far from certain and the boundaries of specialist palliative care are rather blurred, the concept of 'continuity of care' is no easier to define. In the first chapter we attempted to define continuity in palliative care in some detail, suggesting that key aspects relate to the delivery of care over time and the integration of care between professionals and teams, proposing a dynamic model of longitudinal and cross-sectional continuity in palliative care. Importantly and perhaps more simply, continuity may also be seen as what the patient says it is. Chapter 5, which describes patient and carer experience, suggests that for them continuity is key to care that is integrated, consistent and coherent.

### Complex interrelationships in palliative care

Whatever the exact nature of palliative care, its delivery is clearly complex. Its holistic focus should give equal attention to physical, psychological, social and spiritual domains, which demands that it is best delivered in a multidisciplinary manner by professionals with diverse skills. High levels of clinical need in a potentially rapidly changing situation necessitate professional help to be available in and out of normal working hours. Patients being cared for at home, in hospital, hospice and nursing home require that healthcare professionals from primary care, medical and surgical specialities and specialist palliative care are aware of each other's role for each individual patient. This is only achieved if professionals have an understanding of local organisational structures, the primary role of each team and the constraints organisational structures place on individual clinical practice. Professionals must also work to maintain open communication between various teams and understand where the gaps in service delivery are likely to lie. In addition, palliative care works best when professionals have a willingness to cross normal working boundaries in order to fill gaps in care. For instance, the GP who is willing to put up a syringe driver for a patient if the district nurse is not available provides a personalised service that may well make a patient feel highly valued and cared for. Glimpses of such practices are described in Chapter 5.

It might be helpful to reframe the analysis given above and examine different levels of operation when considering continuity in palliative care. At the individual patient level, care needs to be well planned with attention to detail for continuity in terms of relationship, information and management. The patient, however, is embedded within the context of his or her family and other immediate social relationships. Continuity similarly needs to be maintained for individuals and groups close to the patient. Care for the patient and family 'meshes in' with the activity of the professionals and teams caring for the patient. There might be several of these, for example from primary care, from the disease site speciality area and from specialist palliative care. These teams overlap as they care for the individual patient, but they are also part of wider healthcare organisations, which may be institutionally related or diverse (e.g. PCT, acute trust, voluntary hospice, etc.). The individual teams in their organisations will operate within the wider healthcare system at a local, regional or sub-regional network and national level. All of these systems from the patient up to the national level have indistinct boundaries and are continuously changing and evolving. Changes at one level will have an effect at another, such that no part of the whole can be isolated and 'engineered' without ultimately affecting the whole system.

### Continuity of care in palliative care

The models of care, examples of good practice and evidence of failure in achieving continuity of care given throughout this book illustrate how palliative care is delivered within a complex healthcare context. What is good practice in one situation may not be at all effective in another. What was available at one time may not be available at a later date. Conversely, what was provided originally by one provider may later be duplicated by several. In order for continuity of care to be achieved and costly duplication to be avoided, services need to constantly re-evaluate what they deliver, not just within their own field of work and responsibility, but also how they integrate with other services, taking care to ensure that gaps which threaten continuity are not allowed to open up. Models of care need to be evaluated within different contexts to identify strengths and weaknesses, including core aspects that may be transferable to other contexts and alternative methods of implementation. Palliative care is definitely not an area in which a 'one size fits all' solution can be found.

    The experience of patients and their carers in relation to continuity of care is central. If they do not experience consistent, coherent and integrated care at this vulnerable time, their suffering is likely to be increased. Cicely Saunders recognised that personally delivered care is central to the dying patient's needs and Chapter 5 has illustrated this point. Patients do value ongoing personal care and many have identified this as being offered by their district nurse. GPs may be seen as more distant from the patient and barriers could exist to the patient being able to see their GP; for example, difficulty may be experienced in arranging a home visit. It is not possible to make generalisations from this data, since we have only reported studies that were conducted in a few specific areas and that were also highly selective in the patients and carers sampled. Evidence was also presented in Chapter 5 as to how patients might use secondary care, such as the oncology ward, as the focus for receiving personal continuity of care. This seemed to be because patients believed that the oncology ward had up-to-date information about their care, could understand better than primary healthcare teams what their needs were, but also importantly they provided personal continuity.

### Out-of-hours primary care

Great concern is expressed regarding the provision of care out of hours. Personal continuity is almost impossible to maintain for individual patients, although continuity of information is often seen as a good second best. But with personal continuity breached, patients or their carers may endure distress wondering if they should phone the out-of-hours service, if their problems are legitimate, or fear being intensely questioned within a triage system that seems hostile. Some GPs and district nurses (DNs) still do give their personal telephone numbers to dying patients and their carers. Evidence emerged from the Scottish study into experiences of accessing out-of-hours care (Chapter 5) that, even when this happened, patients and carers may be reluctant to use this number, feeling that calling their GP would be an imposition and therefore choosing to call the designated out-of-hours primary care provider.

From this study it also emerged that patient and carer experience of out-of-hours primary care providers was highly variable. Some patients felt that they received excellent care, often expressing surprise when the quality of care exceeded their expectations. Others found the systems in place for triaging calls bewildering and the care received not appropriate or reassuring. Lack of information available for out-of-hours providers about their condition was cited as one reason why they felt vulnerable out of hours. Such lack of information can clearly put professional carers at a disadvantage when attending a patient who is unknown to them. It is, however, most unfortunate when the professional's anxieties are communicated to the patient, in turn leading to fear and distrust of the professional by the patient and carers. This underlines the need for a sensitive approach and good communication skills on the part of professionals, especially those involved in delivering out-of-hours care.

Issues around continuity of information especially into the out-of-hours period has been widely investigated and debated (see Chapter 2). As yet no system exists for sharing of high levels of information between primary care providers and those providing care for their patients out of hours. Patient-held records (PHR) require a high degree of coordination and dedication from both patients and health professionals, which is difficult to achieve and therefore PHR probably at best provide an incomplete record (see Chapter 12). IT systems may provide a solution to providing such information (see Chapter 13) but as yet such systems are not generally available. Issues of connectivity and security of personal data with such systems remain unresolved. Also, since healthcare providers in general are not used to recording high levels of detail about patients on computer, a cultural shift in clinical recording would be needed to ensure adequate information regarding patients is available.

The most effective method of giving out-of-hours primary care providers information regarding patients is considered to be transferring clinical details by fax (or perhaps email) by the GP to the out-of-hours provider. GP out-of-hours cooperatives have collectively accepted that such systems are important and valuable, and should be in place in all co-ops. The practice is also highlighted in the Gold Standards Framework for Palliative Care (GSF) (Chapter 11). However, it can be difficult for practitioners to predict when it is necessary for such information to be made available and information can become rapidly out of date. Evidence suggests that, while many systems are in place for handover forms to be sent, in practice such contact can be patchy. As a result, systems for sharing information cannot be a reliable substitute for out-of-hours providers being skilled in taking a clear history from the patient and using professional experience and expertise in coming to a reasonable and effective management decision.

General practitioners do have the skills for providing care in less than ideal situations where information is limited, the clinical situation is deteriorating and patients and their carers are anxious, as illustrated in Wendy-Jane Walton's personal view (Chapter 3). Recent changes in out-of-hours provision, with fewer GPs being part of such a service, may be problematic for the delivery of palliative care in some areas. Developments are at an early stage and outcomes of these changes are either unknown or speculative. It is important that research is undertaken in monitoring developments so that examples of good and effective practice can be shared and problems identified and avoided.

It will also be important to monitor the impact of using NHS Direct as a central point of contact on palliative patients accessing support out of hours. Early indications have been that NHS Direct does not offer a robust and effective service for palliative care patients. Refinements of the service may allow more appropriate development. For instance the COMPASS helpline [see www.kingsfund.org.uk/funding/partners_for_health_in_london/endoflife_care.html (accessed March 2007)], currently being piloted by NHS Direct in Southeast London, provides information on services and support for patients, carers and healthcare professionals, and may well point the way for future service development. However, other important developments also need to be considered, for example providing palliative care patients with bypass numbers to gain speedy access to the right sort of help and support.

The National Institute for Health and Clinical Excellence (NICE) guidance on supportive and palliative care has called for the availability of DN teams over 24 hours for palliative care patients or access to other nursing care. While 24-hour DN cover is provided within some Primary Care Trusts (PCTs), a resistance to implement this by all PCTs continues and in areas where there are shortages of staff this is likely to be the case across other organisations with little likelihood of substitution. A whole-systems approach to out-of-hours care needs to take particular account of the needs of palliative care patients by introducing linked provision across a number of providers. The increasingly prominent role played by DNs in palliative care provision (see Chapter 4) suggests a way forward to improve personal or relational continuity both within and out of hours.

### The Gold Standards Framework (GSF)

The centrality of the primary care team in delivery of palliative care has been firmly placed on the NHS agenda by the emergence of the GSF. This programme, which stresses the importance of relational, informational and managerial continuity, and facilitates the delivery of these aspects, has been embarked upon to date by around 30 per cent of primary care teams nationally. Evidence emerging from the evaluation of early phases of the GSF suggests that primary care teams feel their ability to deliver palliative care is enhanced through participation in the framework. Whether systems such as the GSF can facilitate palliative care provision in the majority of practices is as yet unknown and the evidence will only emerge with time. However, in a complex environment, the knock-on effects of participating in such developments as the GSF, Liverpool Care Pathway or Preferred Place of Care Tool are also unknown. Such initiatives may well enhance awareness of roles and responsibilities, and patterns of communication, as has the Department of Health-funded national palliative care education programme for district and community nurses. Such initiatives can foster improved collaboration and continuity of care in indirect ways.

### Continuity in a changing health service

Guidelines, care pathways, frameworks for good practice and networks for strategically planning whole services all aim to provide good-quality palliative care including continuity of care. However, whilst achieving continuity in a health service that was relatively stable might have been a challenge, achieving it in a rapidly changing situation is especially difficult. Constant reorganisation within the NHS potentially confounds planning and delivery. Guidelines and frameworks do not function in isolation and cannot be put into practice or made to work like running a machine or an assembly line. They need to work within a network of relationships in complex and overlapping organisations. Pathways for the palliative care patient cannot be simplified as might be possible for patients receiving surgery for a hernia or a cataract. However, the majority of developments within the NHS, particularly 'Payment by Results', seem to be aimed at simplification and streamlining, whilst foundational aspects such as personal continuity by general practitioners are being eroded. In all complex systems changes will have unforeseen consequences. For example, initiatives aimed at improving access to care such as being able to see a GP within 48 hours can mitigate against access in other ways, such as when patients wish to book an appointment in advance at their convenience, as was illustrated to the discomfort of the British prime minister during the 2005 general election campaign.

Primary and community health care is undergoing a major review which might change its nature radically. The white paper *Our Health, Our Care, Our Say*, published in January 2006, and the document *Commissioning a Patient-Led NHS*, published in July 2005, both herald perhaps the widest reform of services in the NHS in its 60-year history. PCTs are to become organisations for the support of Practice-Based Commissioning (PBC) and community services are to be delivered by organisations that can include those from the independent and voluntary sector in addition to NHS Trusts. Whilst the NHS has experienced a limited purchaser/provider split before, previous NHS reforms have largely involved administrative changes at a regional and local organisational and institutional level. Those elements involved in the provision of direct patient care have tended to *evolve* more slowly in response to these changes, clinical need, funding and other resource constraints.

The most recent reforms occurred with the creation of Primary Care Groups (PCGs) in 1999, which transformed into PCTs from 2000 with the amalgamation of health authority and community trust provider functions. This led to a degree of inertia in developments at the service delivery level as the new organisations took time to function effectively. Future changes may more radically affect care provision with the fragmentation of provider organisations and the possibility of private companies vying for different aspects of primary and specialist care provision, leading to the dislocation of formal and informal caring networks. This will affect the relationships between professionals and teams, and may have wide-ranging effects on the delivery of integrated care for patients with the most complex needs.

Many of the features that allow palliative care continuity to be achieved are related as much to such informal networking between staff and teams as to pathways and guidelines, however important these might be. Good communication between health and social care professionals is essential for effective provision of services and where this breaks down, for whatever reason, provision of care can be compromised. Future changes could therefore adversely affect the drive towards achieving integrated and seamless care.

Since this book was conceived the new GP contract was introduced with its direct effect on out-of-hours primary care and refocusing of service provision in terms of the Quality Outcomes Framework (QOF). Many GPs and community nurses believe these changes, enacted clearly for the benefit of providers rather than patients, have been detrimental to the provision of palliative care both by night and by day. The effects of these changes are becoming apparent and associated with increased numbers of complaints (according to defence organisations), many associated with lack of continuity of care. With even more radical changes likely to be put into place within a short timescale, many more examples are likely to emerge.

The central theme set out in this book: the importance of continuity in palliative care with attention to the complexities involved will, however, still be relevant despite all of these health service reforms. Palliative care provision may change radically and there must be uncertainty over its future direction. Clinicians, strategic planners and commissioners will all need to develop systems in response to these changes within the NHS, building on what has been achieved, having vision for the future and at times trying to predict what changes might occur next to avoid surprises as far as possible. Only in this way will continuity of care for the palliative care patient continue and develop further as a characteristic feature of the British healthcare system.

# Index